the lover within

Henderson has written a ground-breaking and personal text of investigations, not techniques, which is a reinvention of Tantric energetics.

East West Journal

Julie Henderson is a boundary-crosser. From the other side of our customarily imposed limitations on self and energy, she beckons us to cross over in safety—in fact, with pleasure—by expanding our energy body to encompass all of life, both inside and outside the body.

Yoga Journal

Henderson's philosophy of understanding energy cycles and patterns permeates her title and encourages the nurturing and sharing of energy between partners.

Midwest Book Review

the lover within

the lover within

Opening To Energy
In Sexual Practice

julie henderson

STATION HILL

BARRTOWN, LTD.

Published under the Station Hill Openings imprint of Barrytown, Ltd., Barrytown, New York, 12507, as a project of The Institute for Publishing Arts, Inc., a not-for-profit, federally tax exempt, educational organization.

Online catalogue and purchasing: http://www.stationhill.org
E-mail: publishers@stationhill.org

Grateful acknowledgement is due to the New York State Council on the Arts for partial financial support of the publishing program of The Institute for Publishing Arts.

Typeset and design by Susan Quasha
Cover design by Susan Quasha
Cover Photograph by Charles Stein

Library of Congress Cataloging-in-Publication Data
Henderson, Julie.
     The lover within : opening to energy in sexual practice / Julie Henderson. – Expanded ed.
        p. cm.
     Includes bibliographical references.
     ISBN 1-58177-017-0 (alk. paper)
     1. Sex. 2. Bioenergetics. I Title.
HQ31.H4718   1999
613.9'6—dc21   99-26107
                                                                             CIP

Manufactured in the United States of America.

I offer this book with deep gratitude

to Susan Rawlins, poet, editor, and friend,
who turned speech into loving and responsible prose;

to Tony Richardson and Robyn Speyer,
for going into new territory with me;

to all who learn with me.

And, after fourteen years' delay,

for Tarthang Tulku Rinpoche
in belated recognition of the transmission that
seeded this first wedding of somatics and tantra.

Contents

List of Exercises

List of Illustrations

Preface to the Revised Edition of *The Lover Within*

I like this book very much. In fact, I feel like the mother of a much loved child who has grown up quite well, but not as expected. Of course, it's me that has changed. When I was writing *The Lover Within* in 1984, I included in it all the most exciting and helpful and pleasurable things I knew about then. It's not the book I would write now, but fortunately it doesn't have to be. It has its own life and its own value.

What I knew then as new and exciting is now an "ordinary" but vital part of maintaining my well-being in everyday life. I am very happy that Station Hill has asked me not only to introduce new people to the book but to add some enticing tidbits of things I have learned since.

For people—and there are many—whose experience of energy and presence is more familiar and convincing to them than the sensations of being a body, this is a good book. It can be particularly beneficial for people who have been led to believe that their perceptions are bad or crazy. It isn't true. It isn't even uncommon to perceive in terms of pattern and flow. Many great artists and athletes describe their most satisfying accomplishments in these terms.

Many people see or hear or sense, at least occasionally, in a range beyond what is usually called "normal." Most of us, in fact, perceive in a broader range of experience than the one we bark our shins against. Mostly, though, since it isn't admitted to be normal, we may deny or suppress our access to this information. *The Lover Within* has the virtue of speaking openly about the possibilities of extended perception in a relaxed and ordinary way. This means that people can get on with "seeing things that aren't there"—or hearing them or sensing them or tasting them or smelling them—with some playfulness and discipline rather than with the bother of worrying about their mental health, at least on the grounds of their extended perception!

For people who long for an experience of sex that is also an embrace, the keys are here.

For people who want to free themselves from the whiplash of habitual reactions to people and situations and their own history, the approaches here can show you how.

For people who love each other but who have lost the energetic "distance" that must exist so that it can be crossed ecstatically, *The Lover Within* offers the real possibility of restoring intensity to love union.

For people who want, at least some of the time, to surrender to the flow of being and aliveness itself, the practices here are an open door.

I sincerely hope that many of you will walk through the door.

Julie Henderson
Napa, California
Schloss Rastenberg, Austria
Gut Helmeringen, Germany

the lover within

1
Origins of the Affair

In introducing a book to the reader, it is customary—and also a courtesy—to indicate its place in the greater geography of ideas. In the case of *The Lover Within*, a very great deal of what is presented arises out of the whole context of my life so that we are faced with the description of a larger than usual context. A bigger piece of the map is needed—the general outlines of California, say, rather than details of Orange County—than if *The Lover Within* were a consideration and testing of a subsection of an established intellectual countryside.

We are caught between overdoing it one way: bringing in references to everything that ever pushed me in this direction; and overdoing it the other: announcing that there *are* no books on this subject and therefore no *written* context to refer to.[1] One approach is ponderous; the other, ignorant and ungenerous.

I have considered including as landmarks in this general map
* the contribution of my professional training as a bioenergetic analyst, and therefore of the whole context of somatics and somatic psychotherapy;
* the influence of my training as an actress and director in theatre;
* other professional training in psychotherapy, such as transactional analysis and Gestalt therapy;
* the whole approach to altered states of consciousness partly described—but largely only indicated—by Milton H. Erickson, M.D.;
* meditative views of consciousness and being (including tantra); and
* sexology, especially what led me ultimately to set aside much of what I had been taught about sex and how it is and should be and what it's all about.

The more I reflected on the issue of context—by what roads and following what signposts did I come to this place?—the more I found myself relying on a few basic concepts. Some of these, I realise, can and do stand there looking a little bald without their own contexts of research and experience.

Probably the most basic assumption I make, and perhaps the

most startling to some people, is that life itself is a form of energy. Do you boggle? The argument for this position is presented in Chapter 6. There is a corollary to this assumption on which much of bioenergetics and other forms of somatic intervention rest, and that is that the body and mind do not exist separate from each other but form a functional unity which meaningfully expresses that life energy.[2]

The second assumption may seem equally alien to some though it is unavoidable in the implications of modern physics and its emerging world view. In our context this view would state that the boundaries you experience between yourself and another, though felt, are not real at the level of energy.[3] Those "boundaries" have to do with variations in the distribution and density of energy rather than actual separation. Investigating the implications of this idea in the context of somatics and psychotherapy, I have found that we can learn to experience our felt boundaries differently than early conditioning prompts us to. The scholarly support for this assertion (and experience) comes from such disparate corners as Buddhist psychology and quantum mechanics.

The third major theoretical landmark is that sensations (including the spectrum of sensations identified as emotions or feelings) can be seen as wave phenomena of this life energy, that such sensations demonstrate the properties of waves in their propagation and movement, and that, like other waves, they can be modified. I think this particular formulation is mine, and here I state it in what can be loosely called bioenergetic or biophysical terms. For me, however, the idea that we can learn to alter what we feel originates in theatre.[4] Theatre training introduced the idea, Gestalt exercises enhanced it, bioenergetics gave it reality and power, meditation allowed equanimity and control.

An important corollary to this is that our various states of mind and emotion, though both volatile and tenacious, are modifiable. There are as many attitudes and approaches to this concept—and goal—as there are psychologies and psychotherapies. I have been most influenced in this area by somatics, the Ericksonian approach to "hypnotherapy",[5] and meditative psychologies, particularly the approaches of zen and tantra.

Finally, and this is the concept that is central to *The Lover Within,* I suggest that sex is at least as much an energetic act as it is

2

a physical one. I realise that this notion may seem nearly as radical as that life is a form of energy. The practical implications of it are profound; the actual experience, both profound and satisfying. I regard sex as one aspect of a human energetic movement towards union, not as a specialised activity somehow separate from life.[6] What happens to us energetically during courtship, foreplay, and intercourse decides whether we like what's happening or not. I have included several basic texts on sexology in the annotated bibliography, but this view simply does not occur in the current literature on sex. That it does not is one of the main reasons I decided to write all this down.

Notes

1. This is not entirely true. Although there are not (to my knowledge) any other books on the energetics of sexuality and union, there is a whole "secret" tradition of Tibetan Buddhism that is based on the experience of energetic union. A few of the books from this tradition have recently been translated from Tibetan (e.g., *The Divine Madman: The Sublime Life and Songs of Drukpa Kunley* and *Mother of Knowledge: The Enlightenment of Ye-Shes mTsho-Rgyal*), but they are not practically useful without a teacher. To say, "The Vajra of the Yab joined the Lotus of the Yum, and together they entered a state of great equanimity," may be evocative, but it doesn't really help with *how*. (NammKai snying-po, *Mother of Knowledge*, p. 13).

2. Alexander Lowen, Wilhelm Reich, Stanley Keleman, David Boadella, et al., in every book they have written. See bibliography.

3. This idea is most fully discussed in *No Boundaries* by Ken Wilbur.

4. Though theatre training, in the main, is not really adequate to allow full choice.

5. I put "hypnotherapy" in quotes here because, although Dr. Erickson was and is justly famous for his work in medical hypnosis, it seems to me far too small a category for his work overall.

6. In *The End of Sex*, pp. 87–108, George Leonard discusses the recent splitting off of sex from other aspects of being.

4

2
The Body
of the Experiment

Experimental psychology largely still resists the realisation that our picture of the universe is no longer Newtonian but relativistic and quantum mechanical (and still changing). Experimental design concentrates on a clean subject-object division when this is not even theoretically possible.

The design of the experimental apparatus influences the outcome of the experiment. The classic example of this—which we are still trying to incorporate into our relationships with reality—sparked the particle-wave controversy over the nature of the electron in the early part of this century.[1] At the time, our minds insisted that somehow the electron *must* be either a particle or a wave. Now it begins to be conceivable to say that when we observe an electron under conditions X, it behaves like a particle; when we observe it under conditions Y, it behaves like a wave. This is staggering and strikes significantly at the very most basic levels of our previous understandings of existence itself.

In psychology and psychotherapy, especially, the person *is* the experimental apparatus. We, the observers, observe ourselves observed. This cannot be an "objective" act.

I learned what I present here through a series of "experiments in being". Most of them were conducted under the supervision of various training therapists in bioenergetics and other somatic disciplines,[2] but all of them arose from the essential fabric of my life and were not separated from my need to know myself and penetrate the mystery of being. In this sense, the experiment can be described as *tantric* because, according to Guenther, it "begins with and insists on immediate experience."[3] Guenther goes on to say that such a position is "naturally different from [the Western philosophic position] which starts with a hypothesis and remains essentially speculative".[4]

Specifically, this learning is based on my exploration of a kinesthetic intuition of surrender to pleasure and union that had never been satisfied by sex-as-I-was-told-it-was-supposed-to-happen.

I grew up with many of the assumptions about sex common to "good" girls who were teenagers in the 1950's. In my case, this meant that sex was for closeness but not passion or ecstasy; that sex was a price I paid for closeness and touching and approval; that pleasure was something related to what a man did; and that I must never, on any account, look at these assumptions or object to them. So I didn't.

Then along came the 1960's and '70's, and there were lots of apparent changes and some real ones. Women were now encouraged to want pleasure and "have" orgasms, preferably many (and absolutely without difficulty). New guilts arose. Masters and Johnson did their famous studies; there were charts and graphs of what was supposed to happen. Because I was still a "good" girl, I tried it that way, too.

In 1975, I began training as a bioenergetic analyst with the Bioenergetic Society of Northern California (a branch of the International Institute for Bioenergetic Analysis). Bioenergetics and its Reichian cousins deal with sexuality and orgasm as the basis for the "energy economy" of the living body.[5] The capacity for orgasm became the basis for a definition of psychophysical health.[6] A clear distinction was made between climax—a limited genital release, not always even pleasurable—and orgasm—a spontaneous, reflexive, pleasurable redistribution of energy in pulsations throughout the whole body. I had two reactions to this: one, it seemed like a tough act to come up with to "prove" you were healthy (still being a "good" girl); two, it touched deeply into "what my body expected" and hadn't found in the adaptations required by the attitudes of the 50's, 60's, or 70's.

As my study of bioenergetics deepened, there began to be a growing and puzzling gap between my increasing systemic capacity for charge, pulsation, and pleasure, and the fact that my experience of sexuality with my partner remained frustrating.

I took refuge in self-castigation; there must be something wrong with me. I re-read all the books on what-goes-wrong and how-it-spozed-to-be.[7] I became ever more helpful and inventive, trying to interest a partner who was already satisfied with what was happening between us—except that I less and less wanted to "do" that, felt less and less like a "good" girl.

In session after session of training therapy, I would confront "Oedipal issues" and early trauma and how to negotiate with a partner—all quite fruitfully. But none of it changed the basic dichotomy between the trusting responsiveness of my body—the increasing cooperation and unity between conscious and unconscious, mental and physical axes of experience—and the overwhelming sense that something was "wrong" sexually. Something essential was going untouched altogether.

Then, in 1980, two things happened at about the same time. The first event was that, under the guidance of my then training therapist, David Finlay, I decided to take another step into trust. If I, in my so trustworthy and responsive body, felt there was something lacking, maybe there was. If the how-to books weren't talking about it, maybe there was nevertheless still something there to perceive and talk about. I began to turn my attention *directly* (if belatedly, perhaps) to what I experienced, what I liked, what excited me, what satisfied me—setting aside all previous judgments, expectations, and demands.

The second event of that time was the outcome of five years accumulated training and practice in reading emotional/psychological experience in the body. This had led almost imperceptibly to an increased range of perception—kinesthetic, tactile, visual, olfactory, gustatory, auditory. It led also to the direct perception of "life energy" through all of these channels. Almost everyone perceives this energy directly, but most people don't know that they do (mostly because their perception isn't validated). This means that a gap exists in consciousness between the perceived and the awareness of perception. I would guess that this is the gap over which the famous "leap of intuition" takes place. Speaking from my own experience, I can say that, if kinesthetic perception is sufficiently refined, the Jungian opposites of sensation and intuition rejoin—like the Ourobouros serpent Jung was so fond of. A fine enough kinesthetic perception will yield results of perception indistinguishable from intuition. I would guess the same to be true for other sensory pathways.

If you do the kinds of exercises in this book consistently over time, you will certainly begin to notice the signs and effects of energetic movement, or lack of it, through all of your senses. You will feel more, see more, hear more, and so on.

7

For me it was easiest first to feel energy as a variety of proprioceptive and tactile sensations; then gradually I came to be able to see its movement and to taste and smell its "flavours". Hearing it still eludes me, but I've no doubt my ears will gradually open to this range. For some, their ears will give the first access.

What this all means in the context of how I learned about *the lover within* is that along about the time I decided to "re-think" the whole issue of sexual pleasure and satisfaction, I was also in a position to perceive what I was missing. I noticed that when my lover penetrated me physically, he didn't penetrate me energetically. The current of his excitement and aliveness remained within him. I felt untouched. Because of all I had learned—much less from books than from a forced return to experience itself—I could no longer split myself off from what I was experiencing and try to make it what I *should* be experiencing. I could no longer mislead myself about what was happening. I was no longer a "good" girl.

I tried sharing this new understanding with my partner, and sometimes the old pattern would change; but basically, he was not interested, and so we parted.

Since that parting, I have continued learning through personal experiment about the voluntary movement and distribution of energy.[1] I learned it in much the same ways and in much the same sequence that I am suggesting to the reader here. Some of the exercises I have invented; some are basic to bioenergetics and other similar disciplines; some I learned from other people and modified. As far as I know, this book is the only place these exercises are discussed and utilised for the purpose of enhancing union, for voluntary energy distribution, for energetic choice in the experience of relationships.

I have done all of these exercises many, many times myself and have explored them with several thousand people in the safe environment provided by training and therapy workshops I have given over the last seven years in the United States, Europe, Australia, and New Zealand. I was the original "locus of experiment" in the investigations of being that led to *The Lover Within*. However, of the thousands of people who have done some or all of this work under my supervision, by far the majority confirm that the exercises work—and work in the ways described. They confirm that they can (and do) learn to merge or separate energetically with a partner as they choose; they report that this gives them a greater freedom, wholeness, and safety individually and in the relationship. They confirm that the same skills allow the break-up of a relationship to complete itself with less of the troubling sense of loss-of-self that usually afflicts at least one partner. They report increased available energy—for sexual union, if they choose—and less frustration by the binding of energy genitally. They say they experience greater pleasure, greater trust, greater capacity for surrender to being.[9]

Notes

1. Heinz Pagels, *The Cosmic Code,* pp. 73-75, 118-122. Many other discussions exist.

2. With respectful thanks and gratitude to Robyn Speyer, Tony Richardson, David Finlay, Jane Loebel, David Boadella, Stanley Keleman, Renato Monaco, Alexander Lowen, Thomas Hanna, Richard Heckler, among others.

3. H. V. Guenther, *Tibetan Buddhism in Western Perspective,* p. 36.

4. *Ibid.*

5. Wilhelm Reich, *The Function of the Orgasm*, pp. 187-194, and others following him.

6. *Ibid.,* p. 59.

7. Thanks for *spozed* to James Herndon in *The Way It Spozed To Be.*

8. I am currently consulting with researchers at the Human Interaction Laboratory, Langley Porter Neuropsychiatric Institute, University of California at San Francisco, in experiments on the voluntary accessing of emotions, including ecstasy.

9. For those who come to this discussion already familiar with such concepts as character structure, I would like to say specifically that I am aware that this approach to (and this experience of) sexuality and union reflect my own character and structure. In the course of eleven years of active training and exploration in bioenergetics, I have learned that there is no one of Lowen's structures—schizoid, oral, masochistic, psychopathic, and rigid—in which I do not significantly participate. However, if life and its designs press me hard enough and fast enough, I will still have a basically schizoid defense reaction. I have the advantages of my disadvantages, however; and I hope that this book reflects them. Most books on sexuality are written by "rigids". All structures, however amiable, suggest their own limits of perception and experience. My work with myself and others suggested it was time something was written about sexuality and union from an alternate perceptual "reality".

10

3
Getting Started

Musicians do *it* with rhythm. Cavers do *it* dirty. Paramedics do *it* repeatedly and until exhausted. Politicans try to control *it*.

What is this *it* that we do and are apparently so obsessed with doing? What is it that is happening that makes *it* so pleasurable when *it is* pleasurable and so frustrating when *it* is frustrating? There are hoards of sex books about how to do *it* so that pleasure is assured, and yet is it ever? Is *it* really a matter of the proper insertion of Tab A into Slot A? or pressing Button B? or Buttons CDE in proper sequence?

Some recent research[1] into passionate love and sexual desire quite convincingly indicates that nearly everybody is miserably frustrated in their longing *and* thinks everybody else is satisfied.

But what is satisfaction? And what specifically needs to happen for you to be satisfied?

I am hoping that one of the things this book offers you is the beginnings of a new language to negotiate satisfaction, to facilitate actual union. I hope that in your relationships, of whatever sex, you can have a language to talk about what you are experiencing. I hope that you and your partner can come to some sort of mutual satisfaction or understanding and don't end up each feeling that the other is just mean.

Sexual experience, the experience of sexual pleasure, varies from person to person. Needs vary from person to person. People assume that what they like is what somebody else likes, that how they experience certain kinds of touching is the way someone else does. All these assumptions need to be questioned.

This book is also concerned with giving you access to certain information and experience not taught in the schools or mentioned in the manuals: how to gain a measure of choice over what happens to your sexual energy. Specifically: how to move it; how to collect it; how to heighten it; how to disperse it; how to share it; how to discharge it—to your satisfaction.

In more technical terms, the book applies information about *voluntary energy distribution* to sexual needs and interests. It is concerned with how to learn to take your energy and direct it into effective patterns within you and in relationship. It's meant to be practical and is full of exercises you can do on your own or with a partner. They are exercises for the physical body, for the energy body, for the mind, and for the will. If you practice them with attention and a kind of respectful playfulness, you can learn something about choice and energy that will apply to every area of your life.

I would like people to have access to this information because it's important to an understanding of what happens between lovers. Many of the troubles that occur between lovers occur because they don't understand that the primary attraction, the primary process, is an *energetic* process

- that is mediated through the body (when the lovers are physical lovers),
- that intercourse is not necessary for the experience of union or of orgasm,[2] and
- that intercourse often occurs without union.[3]

Because people don't recognise these things or, recognising them, don't know what to do about them, confusion follows confusion, and resentment is close behind.

People also aren't aware that they have energetic habits. They don't know if they have a preference for being separate or for being merged, or the preference of their partner; but they may spend their whole lives suffering the results.

Usually, because of conditioning, there is a cultural preference on the part of males for being separate energetically. They are often frightened of union, of feeling soft and melting and merged. Even when they do merge, they stereotypically want to get separate again speedily, as if nothing had happened. Sit up and light a cigarette, etc. Women, on the other hand, are often encouraged to be in a state of perpetual energetic merger with a partner (and to feel that there's something wrong when that's not happening). It helps them to be attentive and aware of another's feelings—which is stereotypically part of their role. But if you are in a relationship with a person who has only the skills of separation and is frightened of merger, and you yourself have a preference for merging and don't really know how to separate, both of you can get into some phenomenally sticky situations, with both people feeling unloved and either abandoned or trapped. Again and again and again.[4] Whereas with even a minimal understanding of the exercises that-teach you how to create your own energetic boundaries, and how to merge and separate energetically at will, you can avoid a lot of that turmoil or better negotiate it.

Sometimes the teacup breaks, and people separate their lives. Often there is great pain involved. In the language you will learn here, I would say that this is the pain of physical separation without energetic separation. Chapter 10, "Union and Separation", discusses this problem and introduces exercises to use to overcome it. Using these exercises, a good deal of unnecessary pain can be avoided or moved through more rapidly and cleanly than usual.

As people learn to unite with themselves within, to allow themselves that pleasure in their own being, then when they do unite with someone else, they can do it out of a respectful desire rather than a sense of starvation. Then the union can be playful and creative—a blessing rather than a dependency.

I will be talking also about another thing that happens when two people come together for purposes of intercourse or making love. They do so usually because there is a strong energetic charge—experienced as excitement[5]—between them. They come together, and the charge is released—the energy is re-distributed—in orgasm. After that, they separate again, both physically and energetically.[6] In the general course of things, if people are together a lot of the time and come together often, there will be less and less charge—less force of attraction—between them because they will be more and more alike energetically. There is less and less dipole moment, as the physicists say; less and less pressure to spark across the gap.

It's possible—this I sometimes call re-inventing sex—to create energetic distance deliberately (when you want to) in order to build charge. This means you can turn up the boost when you want to. Then it becomes a matter of choice and awareness, and of course, some people aren't interested in that; they prefer an accidental magic. But if you want to, you can learn how to build charge at will, partly through learning exercises for energetic separation and union, and partly through other exercises that build charge. Sex between people who know and do these exercises will be more exciting and more satisfying than is usually the case as time passes.

What you can learn from the exercises in this book is gradually to be able to contain higher and higher levels of charge within a relaxed organism, higher and higher levels of energy without contracting. That means being able to experience more and more pleasure—in sex, and in being. You can have a lot of charge in your physical system *without* being relaxed, and that's very uncomfortable; or, you can have too little charge to allow reflexive surrender to pleasure, which is very frustrating. Either energetic condition when added to being dependent on other people for your satisfaction (not *sharing* satisfaction, but *depending* on somebody else for it) creates a lot of the sexual misery people experience.

Notes

1. Presented at the regional conference of the American Association of Sex Educators, Counsellors, and Therapists, Honolulu, October, 1983.

2. To put it another way, union or orgasm can be experienced within the person or between two people without intercourse.

3. Whether that fact leaves you feeling safely separate or frustratedly untouched depends on your own energetic habits and needs.

4. This is not the only possible combination of preferences leading to misery. See Chapter 11, "The Energetic Embrace", for a fuller discussion and exercises for enjoying more options.

5. It also happens, of course, that people come together for comfort, or out of boredom, or in the *hope* that excitement will arise between them.

6. Though, as indicated previously, one of the people may never quite merge, and the other may never quite separate.

4
Energy and Charge:
A First Exercise

Let's look at what I am talking about here when I say "energy" and "charge". For some people, I know, it's still a question whether there is such a thing as "life" energy. For my purposes, I am talking about energy, first of all, in the physical definition: the capacity to do work. That has many manifestations: chemical energy, heat, light, electricity, etc. Each of these forms of energy has an impact on its environment. When I refer to energy in this book, I am talking about the force that has to do with *being,* an energy of aliveness. It is energy in this physical sense: that it has the capacity to do work. When it is no longer present, the physical system is no longer animated, even though other energetic processes continue in the body for some time. That aliveness, that quality of *being* is the energy I'm talking about.

I will be talking in terms of how it arises in the body, how it is restricted in the body, how it extends beyond the body, and how we can move it around. The importance of the exercises is that they help us to rearrange ourselves energetically more to our satisfaction.

"Charge" simply refers to the amount of this energy present in the system, whether overall or localised. It describes the level of energy is a system, as apart from the emotional flavour of the charge, i.e., whether we call it anger, annoyance, or rage depends on the charge. The intensity, not the flavour. Sexually, low charge leads to boredom, lack of desire, ho-very-hum.

EXERCISE 1: This exercise to introduce you to charge is at once very basic and quite advanced. You could repeat it at any level of learning and still benefit.

Either with a partner you trust, or by yourself, come to as high a condition of charge as you can, including your genitals, without climaxing and without tensing your muscles. (Tensing is also called *contracting;* see Chapter 8.) Specifically, if you are masturbating, come to a point of charge, of excitation, just a shade this side of orgasmic inevitability, then stop and wait for an hour—again without contracting physically, emotionally, mentally. Be relaxed and surrendered. Turn your attention to the energy in your body (and beyond your body, if you like) and allow that energy to move as freely as you can. Lie still, or move. Make sounds, sing, dance. After an hour, continue to climax if you wish to.

In this exercise, in addition to charging the genitals, you are inviting an increase in the overall energy level of your being. What raising the energy level, and then pausing and waiting for a time at that level, does is to stretch your own capacity to contain charge. That means you can be more pleasurably excited sexually for a longer time before the reflex of orgasm; the orgasm itself will be more ecstatic.

I remember a person in a group in Australia once asking, How could you *stand* that? as if walking around with all that energy moving in me must be a torture. It certainly would be if I were to contract, to clamp down on the energy. Whereas, if I relax and let it move, the energy stretches me in a way that may itself become orgasmic. I can stretch my energetic limits; I can become accustomed to containing more energy by remaining charged *and* relaxed while postponing discharge. If I do that, I can move to higher and higher levels of excitement and pleasure.

Sometimes, it's true, people do not experience high charge as pleasurable; they experience it as discomfort. Those for whom high charge is uncomfortable usually experience sex less in terms of pleasure than as a way to relieve inner pressure. They don't want to spend much time—or any time—increasing that pressure, which is the way they would experience any heightening of their energy level. They want to discharge (or repress) what has already accumulated. They're often interested in having intercourse frequently—briefly, but frequently—to keep the systemic energy level relatively low. (You'll hear this refered to frequently as "Wham, bam, thank you, m'am"—or the female equivalent, though I know no expression for it.) Given our cultural attitudes and upbringing around sexuality, it may be that this kind of experience is the usual. The idea of allowing charge to build up over a fairly long time, or deliberately building charge without immediately discharging it, may seem a strange idea to many people. The fact of the matter is, it's uncomfortable for some because they are at the limit of the energy they can systemically *contain* (in the technical sense, see the fuller discussion on pages 42–44). Of course, it's relative: what's high for me may be low for you. But we can each stretch and expand the amount of energy we can hold while remaining relaxed; we can create a kind of energetic tonus that allows more and more intense experiences of surrender, pleasure, and satisfaction.

This exercise brings us up again and again to the limit of what we can *now* contain (without discharging) and asks us to stay there, relaxed, for some time.[1] The energy is still in the sytem whether or not we are even aware of it. During the pause, the energy may disperse away from the genitals, bringing the whole body to a higher energy level. Later, if you do decide to carry on to climax, you will be starting over, but from a base line that is higher than the energy level you usually start from. The energy is there in your system, so when you draw it again into your genitals, it will be drawing with it more energy from the whole of you, and since you now have a bit more capacity, you'll go up higher than before. That means that gradually you can spend more and more time at higher and higher energy levels, pleasurably. After some practice (*not* mechanical, not Tab A into Slot A), this can develop into an experience called *dwelling in the valley of orgasm.*

Notes

1. Keep in mind that you are very likely to read this exercise hearing what you expect to hear from life—even though it's only me. For example, when my colleague, Ginny Elliott, read the description of this exercise in first and second drafts, both times she heard "*Hold* this energy for one hour", and, as she said, immediately collapsed her energy field both times. What a job of work all that holding would be. I am only suggesting that you move to this higher level of energy and rest there—no effort, no holding. Let life do it. See Chapter 8, "The Energetic Breaths", for a description of energetic collapse.

5
Confusions of Love

Personally I get nervous reading so many pages about sex with no mention of love. Love is a mystery, surrounded by a thousand peripheral definitions. In a way, this book is almost entirely concerned with love—with the pains we suffer looking for it, with the confusions that exist about what it is, with a movement towards more conscious loving.

I can say that love is a mystery; I can even list many of the thousand definitions. Still, you are likely to "know" already what love is; you may even resent it if I say you are confused about it.

Fact of the matter, it's my job now to confuse you—just a bit—to dislodge your preconceptions about love and let them shift and drift until they come into a new resting place. One of my finest teachers—Milton Erickson, M.D., the innovative hypnotherapist— used to say that until you're willing to be confused about what you already know, you can't know anything bigger, better, or more useful.

6

The Energy Body

From an energetic perspective, boundaries are arbitrary and learned. Though we are not separate energetically from the whole, we learn to establish "felt" separations. We can "end" at the skin, or down the block somewhere, or we can retire above the neck, or behind our eyes. *Where* we feel ourselves separate depends on what we have learned. Always the question is: How much choice do you have? Where do you want to live?

First, just conceptually and imaginatively, remember that energy and matter are not different. Matter is a very condensed form of energy. At the level at which that is true, there are no dividing lines, no stopping places, no separateness, no objects—just variations in density. Energetically, then, we don't stop at the skin. It's our cultural assumption that we do, and not all cultures assume it. It's not true at the level of quantum physics, and it's not true experientially. When someone walks up to you, you start feeling "touched" long before he or she gets to your skin. Along about two or three feet away, we begin to feel that other person as dangerously, or rudely, close; they have stepped "inside" of us. That's because we have an energetic skin or boundary as well as our physical skin. The skin of this energy body usually can be felt at the accepted "social" distance of two to three feet, but it can and does with some people extend habitually some twenty or thirty feet.

EXERCISE 2: Notice how your energy body expands and contracts according to situation and event. As you sit and read this, how far do "you" extend? The next time you are in a bank line? Going for a walk through the country? Paying bills? Making love? Is there ever a time when you feel you go on forever? Notice the changes in how much space you take up as you *imagine* bank line, country walk, bills, beloved.

It's this energy body or field that we're going to be learning to move. First of all, it's helpful if you have some direct experience that there really is something there, however mysterious.

EXERCISE 3: Take your hands and rub them together vigorously, making sure you get the fingers and thumb and top and bottom, the whole hand. This "charges" your hands.

Friction is one way of moving energy to the place you want it, in this case to your hands, so that when you stop rubbing, you will have more energy in your hands than when you started. The contrast helps awareness of the *something* there.

Rest. Let your hands drift apart a little bit and feel the space between your hands. Probably you will be able to feel a difference. What do you feel? If you "bounce" the space between your hands lightly, like slowly playing an accordion, the energy will get more dense, and you'll find it easier to feel. Pulsate the energy. One of the things we'll be learning to do is how to bounce or pulsate the whole energy body instead of just the field around your hands. You may feel pressure or tingling or a sense of increased density between your hands, or something that is wholly your own. Whatever sensations are present, that is how you will begin to feel energy; that the Stuff. It's distributed through and around your body, more or less, depending on your habits of distribution.

The Russians say they can now measure that field, and they call it the "Biological Plasma Body".[1] They say it is actually what physicists call a plasma, that is, an electrically neutral, highly ionized gas composed of ions, electrons, and neutral particles. Those particles are so close to being pure energy that, like the electron, they behave as particles or waves depending on the apparatus we use to perceive them.

EXERCISE 4: Assume this is not all crazy. Give an imaginative guess at how far out your field goes. If you don't have a direct sense of it, make it up. How far out from the limits of your skin do you go? Two feet? Three? Two inches? If you sense nothing at all, check outside the room or down underneath the skin of your body. Does your field go further out in front than in back? Up higher than it goes down into the ground?

Your energy body can be dense or diffuse.

EXERCISE 5: Imaginatively check the density of your field. Is it "thicker" than the air outside you? ("You" extend to the edges of your field, remember.) Does it feel thin like mist? Or like a fine web? Does it seem even thinner than the air beyond the field? Within your body, do some places feel denser than others?

Fields also expand and contract.

EXERCISE 6: Check to see what movement there is in your field, as well as how far out you go. Does the field follow your intention? Does it respond to yor wondering what "it" is doing? Imagine an angry gorilla leaping out of the closet at you. (Did your energy move back and in? Where?)

Under optimum conditions, your energy body extends out to a distance that's comfortable for you, is appropriately dense, and expands and contracts gently like a breath. The pulsation of the field produces pleasure as a kind of harmonic of being. All of this varies in specifics according to you and your situation.

Unfortunately, almost nobody functions daily in this way. We've all developed energetic habits, pretty much, so we don't pulsate very much and don't like being alive very much. Most of us. Have you ever had the experience that you have no reason, no excuse, simply to feel good, to feel happy? that some situation has to change first? The pleasure that arises from pulsation needs no reason, only enough trust in the moment of life to allow pulsation to arise.

When someone like Jesus says, "The kingdom of God is within you," he is not joking. Life itself is within you, and always available. It is only a question of learning how to open to it, to relinquish the tight fist that holds you seemingly separate. There are two reasons why this kind of opening is difficult. One, you really do need to learn first to make the boundaries that let you feel separate. But, two, most of us are taught how to do that by people who themselves have never learned the next step, which is to let go of those boundaries and remain aware or to let the boundaries pulse with the movement of the whole in the small. So it happens that in learning to separate we also learn habits that limit our choices.

Notes

1. Sheila Ostrander and Lynn Schroeder, *Psychic Discoveries Behind the Iron Curtain*, p. 202. The bioplasmic body or energy body has 22 references in the index. The principal researchers seem to be V. Inyushin, V. Girschchenko, N. Vorohev, N. Shorisski, N. Fedorova, and F. Gibaldulin. For specific articles, see Ostrander and Schroeder's bibliography.

7

Energetic Habits

Habits are the shorthand of behaviour. You have habits for driving a car. You don't, fortunately, have to think about each move; it would be exhausting and dangerous. Energetic habits arise from the same kind of repeated practice in response to circumstance. As children, we find ourselves in certain situations, which demand or allow a certain range of experience, behaviour, and response. We decide that that's the range that *life* allows (even though it's only Mum or Dad or Aunt Agatha). We get into the habit of responding as if that situation were still current, long after Mum and Dad and Aunt Agatha are no longer calling the shots.

Many people drive cars, the familiar moves revealing their individual styles. Each of us has a "range" of driving behaviour. Some are competent; some are dangerous; some are boring. If your driving is very important to you, you go to high performance driving school, break a lot of lousy habits, and build good ones; your driving goes beyond competence to elegance.

What about sex, then, and life? If you haven't yet learned the full range of what it is to be human, you too can be boring or dangerous, bored or endangered. As you grew up, people and events taught you to restrict the movement of your energy, the life within you. You are hedged in by energetic habits that you know nothing about and that decide what you think life is like. They limit how much of life you can know, how much pleasure you can feel, how passionately you can respond. This is like being given a Ferrari and mistaking it for a '37 Plymouth.

You can learn to have choices about what you're doing with your energy. This includes becoming aware of what your energetic habits are and developing the "energetic muscles" to free yourself from those habits. Voluntary energy distribution is a lot easier than you might think.

I'd like to remind you that you are an energy-producing system. You take in food and you take in air, and in all of your tiny cellular furnaces you oxidise the fuel and create all kinds of energy: chemical energy, mechanical energy, heat energy—as far as we can tell, even some light energy. All of these forms of energy can occur in the absence of life. The cell is somehow also *alive*. The extension of that aliveness into its surroundings we call the *energetic body*. This is the stuff that we're going to be moving around. Moving that energy around in new ways will change the way your body operates, the way your mind operates, the way you experience being.

$E = mc^2$ is an absolutely basic and relevant statement in this context.[1] In 1905 when Einstein formulated his famous equation, he set in motion conceptual shifts, the implications of which are still emerging. Many people reject the implications outright. In the nineteenth century, physics—our way of understanding how things work—was markedly deterministic, and all things were seen as discrete and material. Atoms (if they existed at all) were tiny hard balls that bounced off each other in very Newtonian ways. Living creatures stopped at the skin, each separate and discrete like the atoms. But we live now in the twentieth century, and our physics has expanded into unsettling new territory. We are beginning to experience and describe how things work in much different, more exciting—and often more disturbing—ways.

In a sense that is more real than we can usually get in touch with, there is no stopping place between you and me, between you and the air around you, you and the floor, you and your blissful and aggravating beloved. Of course, each of us experiences separateness. But the way you experience yourself as separate is different from the way I do, different from the way your boss does, your mother does, your lover does. Some people experience their learned separateness similarly to the way I do (or you do), but everybody's experience is different, and everybody's experience is *learned*. When we're born, we do not experience ourselves as separate. Margaret Mahler's researches suggest that the psychological birth of the infant—this learning to feel separate—is a gradual process that normally takes about three years.[2] Some of the most crazy-making things that happen to us occur when we are merged with someone who is not "there" energetically. It can make for a very scary experience of what life is like—intimately and inescapably empty and lifeless. Some people meet this horror very early on, even in the womb. I have a friend and colleague, who arranged (he tells me) to be born prematurely to get out of that situation. That womb was not a good place for him to be.

So, quantum mechanically speaking, each one of us is an energy nexus, an energy density, within the whole. That nexus has more or less awareness—and *that* really is a mystery. As part of our awareness, we learn to create boundaries.

EXERCISE 7: Close your eyes and turn your awareness inward. Notice which parts of your physical self, your body, you can feel. Can you feel your feet? the insides of your feet? Their bones? Ditto your arms, pelvis, legs, mouth, spine? What parts can't you feel at all? What parts are sort of there, like ghosts? Now, where in all this are *you*? When you say, "*I* am feeling my feet," where are you? Where is the awareness that speaks in you coming from?

Most times, people answer this question by saying they hear the voice in their heads. Is that where "you" live? To put yourself in your head creates an arbitrary boundary—a decision has been made that "you" live up there in your skull. That boundary at the neck cuts you off from the greater part of your experience, your feelings, your perceptions, even your mind.[3] This leaves a lot of you uninhabited and unconsidered. A lot of your life is not conscious in you. We build such boundaries in various places throughout the physical body and in the space beyond it. Some we hold very rigidly in place; others we allow to move. You can get in touch with some of the boundaries you build outside your body by recalling how you feel—and what you do—when *another* four people step into the elevator.

Most of us, of course, don't know what our energetic habits are or how they limit us. Some people "are" just behind their eyes, and some are way out the back door somewhere—an "I" that is not in the body at all. Still others are anywhere but in their heads. *All of these are learned boundaries.*

Each of the exercises we do here is an invitation to own the whole space, to inhabit your whole body, to rearrange your learned and limiting boundaries so that you have more space to be—an invitation to occupy all of you.

EXERCISE 8: Pick a room in which you feel comfortable (or pleasurably anticipatory, if you know of such a space). This is the boundary you are about to practice. Stand near the centre of the room (Though later you'll find this isn't necessary, it is helpful in the beginning.) Look the room over to get a sense of the space physically. Now fill it—fill it with *you*. Imagine it, visualise it, say it, sing it, dance it, feel it, *do* it. Whatever helps. When you have filled the space as much as you can for now, begin to bring your energy in and around you like a sphere. Bring it in until you are surrounded by yourself—by your energy body—to a distance of three or four feet. Let the sphere go as far into the ground and up into the air as it goes out to the sides. Notice that as you bring your energy in, it gets denser. You may see it or feel it or hear it or taste it—that's another matter of preference. When you've brought your energy into this sphere, hold it there briefly, "bounce" the edges in and out a bit if you like, then let it go back out again to fill the room. It will be easier this time. Notice the sensations that go with this expansion of yourself into space. Then again bring your energy back in towards your body. Notice that it is even denser than last time. It may begin to push back a bit against the pulling in at some point. Feel that resilience—that push to expand yourself. Hold at that point without contracting; bring the energy in a bit more. Hold, and bounce the edges of your field. Allow the boundary to expand a few inches, then draw in a few inches, then let it out—in and out, like the wings of a bird feathering. Release again into the expansion.

You can repeat this movement as often as you like. Try the same expansion/contraction movement in spaces of various sizes. This gives you a chance to try different boundaries. The more you practice moving your energy—your self—in this way, the easier it will get, and the denser the field you will be able to build.

Aikido offers a variation of this exercise in which the instruction is, "Expand your energy to include all of space and time. Next draw your energy back and bring it in and down to a speck. Disappear the speck. Repeat." This big an energetic "piston" generates a lot of power. Even though it may seem on the face of it an impossible exercise, try it. See how big you can let your universe be, how big you can let yourself be. If you can fill the whole universe of space and time, what separation is there between you and life?

This basic exercise, whether your chosen boundary is the universe or your walk-in closet, does three things. It begins to give you choice over your boundaries; it strengthens your energetic muscles; and it also introduces you to two of the three energetic "breaths"—in-and-out and dense-to-diffuse.

What we're going to do in the next chapter is to look at the ways our energy moves naturally—in and out, up and down, condensing and diffusing—and some of the results of developing restrictive habits about any of these movements.

Notes

1. From further down the path, I hear that *energy* is not always conserved. The world turned for me on this one. Some people are not excited. We may say that *most* of the time mass (i.e., matter) is conserved; nevertheless, the occasions when matter is *not* conserved (as in radioactive decay and nuclear explosions) are certainly central to the dilemmas of our age. If *energy* is not conserved, what is the base/matrix beyond energy? What *is* "conserved"? Some "crazy" physicists are suggesting consciousness itself is the matrix.

2. Margaret Mahler, *The Psychological Birth of the Human Infant*, pp. 52–120.

3. Recent evidence seems to indicate that the "mind"—seen as perceptive intelligence—extends throughout the body and beyond.

8

The Energetic Breaths

There are three basic energetic breaths: in-and-out (expansive/ contractive), diffuse-to-dense, and up-and-down. There are also two basic ways of relating to an "established" boundary which we will look at—containment and compression.[1]

The free flow of energy is a pulsation up-and-down and in-and-out with variations of density. Looking at the flow of energy in and around a lively person is like watching the strong, subtle currents of a river. Taking all the movements together, the flow is spiral, perhaps helical—probably a double helix, going up at the same time it comes down—meanwhile, mind you, diffusing and condensing as needed. This is difficult to visualise and stunning to watch. It's not so hard to *do*, I find. But give a moment to imagining all those "invitations" to helical movement in the DNA itself—minute river interconnected to river, transforming energy and determining flow.

First Breath

Probably the easiest component of this movement to recognise is the in-and-out that is expansion and contraction. For usual social purposes in the United States, most people extend out energetically three or four feet. It's considered the polite distance. Some people, however, habitually place their boundaries farther out or closer in.

EXERCISE 9: Locate your current energetic boundary. If you can't feel it or see it, guess; you'll probably be right. How far out from your skin is it? Is this your usual boundary? Does it change as you ask yourself this question? How do you feel about extending out into space?

As I said, this first breath of energy, this in-and-out movement, is the easiest of all the normally occurring energetic movements to recognise. We are accustomed to expand our energy when we feel good about what's happening. We move out to embrace the event. We contract our energy, usually, when we don't like what's happening—when we want to move away from it. So expanding our energy is usually associated with feeling good, and contracting our energy is usually associated with feeling distant or annoyed or frightened.

31

For most people, movements of energy occur in response to events; however, it's important to understand that the movements themselves produce characteristic feelings. So, if you can learn to expand your energy *even in a situation you don't like*, you can learn to feel good in that situation anyway. Your feelings can be independent of the event (to the extent that you want them to be). It is possible to learn this independence by practising voluntary movement of your energy.

Similarly, in many situations we have the habit of contracting; that produces "bad", unnecessary or uncomfortable, feelings. These exercises let us practise not contracting. A contraction is an unspoken objection. Something happens that we find threatening, and we want to move away from it. If we felt free to, we would move away physically—out of the room, out of the relationship, out of town. Sometimes we can't leave. More often we have been taught we mustn't leave. We have learned to do something else instead. We learned to leave energetically. We learned to contract away from the event even though our bodies are still present. Energetically, we are then more or less absent. Contrast the liveliness of most children (up to a certain age) with the relative lifelessness of most adults.

EXERCISE 10: It is of great value to learn to object to what's happening without contracting, energetically or physically. At first, you may find it quite a puzzling or offensive notion to separate what is happening from your response to it—to allow the event without contracting yourself because you don't like it. You can pick a simple situation you don't like and practise relaxing instead of contracting.

Sit some place comfortable. Think of someone you don't like (Howard Cosell, Donald Duck, your boss). Think of how much you don't like him. Be aware of the parts of your physical body that tighten up *as part of* this dislike. Go on disliking him, and consciously relax the tightnesses. (Use whatever skills you know for relaxation: deep breathing, self-hypnosis, jumping jacks, hollering into a sack.) Dislike him without muscular contraction. Go ahead: object! *and* relax!

Though simple, it's a profound exercise in its effects. You may find in trying it that you feel your "objection" lacks force if you don't contract. Experiment with it anyway.

EXERCISE 11: Consider expanding to *include* the energy of the event within yourself. This has remarkable effects. Forgiveness and mercy are the feelings associated with this particular energetic response. Magnanimity.

Our energy expands and contracts naturally—as naturally as breathing. Often our responses become habitual and limiting. There are people who habitually expand their energy and people who habitually contract it. Letting any one of these perfectly normal movements of energy become a habit has specific negative consequences.

A person who habitually contracts his energy often has cold hands and feet, gets scared frequently, and is a little frightened all the time—an unconscious habit of fear. When we contract too far,[2] we feel afraid, cold, cut off, helpless. People who are in the habit of contracting—who are a little bit contracted all the time—have a hard time saying no,[3] standing up for themselves, objecting, taking up space—all the things that come from an unwillingness (or a feeling that it is not safe) to expand. Usually, they have forgotten how to expand.

It's more difficult to point out the disadvantages of their habit to people who usually expand their energy, but often they do it to avoid being touched by tender feelings or feelings of vulnerability and openness. If we expand too far,[4] we become ungrounded and begin "ballooning"—we feel grandiose or out of touch with other people's needs for space. Being around over-expanded people can be like sitting in the same room with an overstoked furnace. These people use continual expansion like an energetic blaze to keep others at a distance. They need to have a choice, too. The more choice we have over how our energy moves, the freer our responses to life.

Both expansion and contraction are normal—the two poles of a breath. It's important to remember that contraction is just as appropriate as expansion, and that both can be inappropriate at times. You wouldn't choose only to breathe out any more than you'd choose only to breathe in (though some people try). In a neutral situation, the normal energetic breath pulses in and out equally. Then when something happens in our world (inside or out), we like it, or we don't. Unconsciously, we expand towards it or contract away from it. The expansion is a pleasure; the contraction may temporarily aid survival. But one of the things that learning to have choice over your energy distribution can do for you is greatly to increase the number of situations in which you feel willing to expand rather than contracting. A small expansion to include the event (see page 33) gives you more freedom of action. When you contract away from an event—to keep it from touching or influencing you—you limit your options of behaviour. Most people go into a negative trance state in which they experience no choice at all.

You can test your personal and cultural limits about what is "appropriate" to expand towards or into or to contain. That doesn't mean running right out to embrace a rapist. It doesn't mean choosing injury. Even when danger presents itself unavoidably, most of us are not capable yet of being fully present, loving, relaxed, contained, *and* capable of right action. But there are many other situations we are accustomed to finding unpleasant, annoying, angering, frightening, saddening, and so forth; in these situations we can experiment with expanding into life rather than contracting into "no". Having this choice basically means increasing the number of situations in which we are willing to feel in harmony and capable of appropriate, effective action, instead of freezing or exploding.

EXERCISE 12: Repeat the boundary exercise (Exercise Number 8, pages 27–28), this time from the point of view of expansion and contraction. Pay particular attention to how your mood changes as you move your energy in and out. Don't look for a "right" mood change; just focus on what is; each experience will be different. Try also imagining certain situations, "positive" and "negative" ("happy" and "sad"), and notice how your energy moves in response.

Second Breath

The second energetic breath is also in-and-out, but in another dimension: that is, it involves diffusion and condensation. Our habits of diffusion and condensation are usually hard to extricate from our habits of expansion and contraction. In reality these movements are inseparable, and we tease out their components to make things easier to talk about and to visualise. With this in mind, we can talk of the effects of changing density in your field, which can be as fine as mist or as thick as soup.

When you make your energy body dense, it protects you by reducing the influence of other systems "outside". For example, it slows down the impact of other people's feelings as they come at you. If you make your energy dense, it also happens often that people tend to experience you as powerful and charismatic (unless, of course, their field is denser and more flexibly contained than yours).

Diffusing your field sensitises you and strengthens your awareness of "external" events. Diffusing your field also increases empathy—that is, feeling other people's feelings as your own. If you don't know that what you are feeling belongs to someone else, it can be quite confusing and upsetting. People sometimes diffuse their fields specifically in order to figure out what other people are feeling, especially when they aren't permitted to ask. Like almost every energetic habit, this one is formed in childhood. For example, if four-year-old Charlie lives with a mother (or a father or . . .) who insists that "everything if fine" while handing out unexpected thunderbolts of punishment and conflicting responses to everyday situations, Charlie will learn the habit of diffusion in order to find out the truth he needs to survive. Since we can never be 100 percent sure that our guesses are right, this diffusion in order to "psych out" other people can also lead to anxiety or paranoia. But when you are with people you like and trust, your choice to diffuse your field and merge with them, to become one energetically,[5] creates a whole range of pleasurable feelings, from comfort to bliss to ecstasy. Under some circumstances, most people diffuse in this way without thinking—taking a walk through the woods in spring, for example.

Despite the pleasures of diffusion, it isn't a great *habit* to have. Like habitual contraction, habitual diffusion (especially an habitual expanded diffusion) makes some things in life difficult—like feeling separate from other people, like knowing what you feel and what you want, like saying no, asserting an opinion, asking for a raise.[6] The habit is unfortunate in everyday life; to be *able* to do it is wonderful. People who are *unable* to diffuse and merge have other problems, like feeling so separate they can't imagine what love is.

EXERCISE 13: Become aware of density in your field. See or feel or guess how dense or diffuse your field is. It is more dense in front than in back? Or above your head than under your feet? Does the density change as you become aware of it? Do you expand or contract as you observe your energetic body?

A person who habitually diffuses his energy field often has very extended boundaries. His energy drifts thin but far—often as far as thirty or forty feet. Such a person often gets labelled as having "boundary problems". This is not a surprise, since energetically he experiences that other people are walking around inside of him—which is a true perception of what is happening within his energy body. Because his field is so diffuse and expanded, he has little experience of emotional or energetic separation from others and little protection from their energetic impact.

If you want to be at one with the universe, practising simultaneous expansion and diffusion of your field is a good exercise to start with—in a safe place, with people you trust. The danger is a loss of self, a loss of return to separateness.

EXERCISE 14: One half of the Aikido exercise I mentioned earlier (see page 28) is to expand your field until you contain the universe. There is no suggestion, however, that the field need be diffuse. How densely can you fill the universe? The second half of the exercise, the contraction into nothingness, invites a terrific condensation of the field. It's an exercise that builds very strong energetic muscles.

Though diffusion is not a negative thing, there are so many unpleasant consequences of habitual diffusion that I want to mention them again: you find yourself involuntarily empathic (that is, feeling other people's feelings whether you want to or not), subject to feeling the misery of other people as a kind of poison, subject to feeling violated again and again by the everyday activities of other people. It's very common for people with habitually diffuse fields to experience themselves as literally *hit* by other people's strong feelings. That's why their reactions are judged extreme by other people who don't have diffuse field habits.

Diffusers often hear, "Don't take it so hard. Don't be so sensitive. I didn't *do* anything." When you hear that said or say it yourself, it's often because the person in question has a diffuse and expanded field, is energetically merged, and so has no protection—no separateness—from the energetic events going on in another person.

Condensation is usually easiest to learn when boundaries are held close to the body. In the beginning it's easier to experience your field as dense if you collect your field close around you. However, it doesn't really have anything to do with how expanded or contracted you are. You can have a dense expanded field or a diffuse contracted field—as well as the more usual diffuse expanded field or dense contracted core inside the body surrounded by a very finely diffused, expanded "sensing" field.

EXERCISE 15: Repeat the basic boundary exercise. This time give your attention to the process of diffusion and condensation. Notice that the more often you repeat the exercise, the denser your field gets. If you tend to maintain a diffuse field, keep this movement until you feel your energy body dense enough to protect you. This is the "body of light" suggested as a protection or meditation by some mystical schools. Let it be radiant and dense. If condensation is easy for you, move into a larger space and practise diffusing. If no human constriction offers you enough space, move outdoors. Lie on the ground in a field and look up. Spread yourself out into the sky until you can begin to feel what it is to merge. Then return to youself.

There are no particular "practical" disadvantages to an habitually dense field;' that is, in the world-as-it-is, condensation is appropriate. To be stuck in a dense field that is contractive or compressed, however, feels stagnant, trapped and depressed. Again, choice is the key.

Third Breath

The third energetic breath moves up and down, keeping us balanced between depression and exhilaration. Again, people learn habits and preferences within this movement.

On one end, you can "let down" your field. This is something we

37

all need to be able to do; it is the movement that allows us to return to the earth for rest and nourishment. But, if it becomes a habit to let your energy fall, you will experience energetic collapse. The "feel" of this is fatigue and helplessness. This habit—like all others, learned and maintained for reasons of survival—leads to experiencing life as a constant struggle in which you never truly get what you need. Feeling unnourished and helpless, the role you know best is victim. Habitual energetic collapse finally leads to a kind of floppy depression, compensated by an eternal hope and promise to "be good" so that you will be upheld and nourished. Energetically, this habit both arises from, generates, and maintains a situation in which you are not taking in or retaining enough energy to support yourself.

The other half of the "breath" that includes collapse I call "ballooning". This breath draws energy up out of the lower body—off the ground—and is distributed around some portion of the upper body in an unsupported, rather extended, and fairly dense field. People with the habit of ballooning often give the impression of being very energetic, but it's all "up in the air"—usually from the waist or shoulders up. Such people don't have much contact with the ground—that's why I like the image of a balloon with its thin string hanging down to the ground.

As with the other energy movement patterns, this one is very helpful if there are certain things you want to do. (Every one of these movements is necessary and useful.) If you want to observe very carefully, if you want to "keep an eye" on what's happening around you, this movement brings a great deal of energy to your eyes. However, if you hold your energy up in this way over a prolonged period, you will probably end up feeling suspicious.

Ballooning happens spontaneously in a lot of cocktail party flirtations because of the natural exhilaration that follows this movement (in the beginning). Because people who balloon habitually as a defense have a great deal of energy "up" and available for being attentive, they can be great charmers. Or bullies, in another manifestation. Whether charmers or bullies, they live with the expectation that if they don't control what you do, you will control them. From this survival stance, there is not much difference between paying attention and watching out.

Some people are mildly—or more than mildly—ballooning all

the time. They do it because they have experienced that if they are not "on top" of what's happening, if they are not in control of what's happening, "arranging" things all the time, *they* will be arranged, controlled, dominated—to the loss of their integrity as people. So they move their energy up and out in this tippy-toe way to protect themselves. There are very few of us who have not learned a need for this response.

People who habitually collapse their fields are usually very attracted to people who balloon because they are looking for someone to hold them up. It's easy to see, though, that this kind of interaction is supported—insisted on really—by the myths of our culture: the clinging flower and the tower of strength are difficult roles to escape. People who learn to balloon are attracted to their role as tower, bask for a time in this projection of perfection, and say whatever the drama demands: "You are the moon and stars. I will never leave you," etc. But this posture is impossible to maintain on either side, so ultimately the ballooner cuts the string and goes off, Pfffffluuufffp! Into the sunset, but not hand in hand. (I would advise, whether you are charmer or charmed, pay attention to what is *done* rather than *said* on either side. Whether you offer the moon or expect it, you'll end up looking astonished or aggrieved if you depend on delivery.)

EXERCISE 16: Pick a room you like to be your arbitrary boundary. Fill it with your energy body, but only from the waist up. How do you feel? Then try it from the shoulders up. And from the neck up. From the eyes up. What sensations and feelings go with these extremes of ballooning? Experiment with varying the density of your field as you "keep on top of things". You may want to try contracting your field as well as holding it up. Do any of these energy distributions feel suspiciously familiar? Or particularly comfortable?

EXERCISE 17: Now fill the space again, expanding to fill it only from the waist down. What do you experience? How do you feel in your upper body? If you can, let your energy drain down, or run down, diffusing into the ground. How do you feel? Now lower your energetic boundary even more, displacing your energy below your hips, then below your knees. What effects do you experience? Experiment with a diffuse field and then a dense one. Do you feel "at home" with any of these distributions? Does a familiar sense of fatigue or loneliness or abandonment begin to creep over you? Possibly you can't wait to shake off this distribution and get back to one you like. If so, notice how you do it and what you like.

There is a big difference between losing your energy through a habit of collapse and having a consistent energetic connection with the earth (being "grounded"). One leads to fatigue, the other to a sense of security and confidence.

EXERCISE 18: To experience the difference, first repeat Exercise 17 to remind yourself of the sensations of energetic collapse; then gather your energy together in a comfortable, fairly dense sphere. Let the sphere extend a few inches into the ground. Be aware of what you experience. Move around while maintaining this energetic expansion into the earth. Does walking this way feel any different to you? Then, standing or walking, let your field become subtly denser below the navel than above it. What sensations arise? Is your sense of yourself in relation to people or objects in the room any different?

This is quite an advanced exercise, so don't be concerned if you need to practise it many times to feel any effect. If you want more along these lines, any warm-up exercises from T'ai Chi are designed to assist this process of grounding.

Holding Your Breath

There is another energetic movement, an effort like a *held* breath, which I call compression. Compression is the result and cause—it is very much chicken-and-egg to decide on its origins—of most chronic depression. When your field is fairly dense, fairly contracted, and you sit on it—sit on yourself, really—you have created a compression. There's a push down and a pull up simultaneously.

EXERCISE 19: To experience the effects of compression, do a number of jumping jacks—not so many as to exhaust you, but enough that your pulse is up and you are breathing more rapidly. Stand, take a few normal breaths; then contract your anus, clench your jaw, and tighten your shoulders. You may want to jump right out of this (or you may find it oddly comforting), but stay with it long enough to notice the sensations that arise between your neck and pelvis. Then shake it off, dance around a little, and make some noise to free yourself.

People do this in order to endure. It's great for that; this habit, especially if prolonged, gets very uncomfortable.

For me, there is no other energy distribution that has such a bad taste. It's associated with feelings of guilt and unworthiness, or resignation to burdens, of having the world on one's shoulders, of having to go on and on without respite in the mantle of martyrdom. Given my preferences, I would *only* choose this distribution if I had exhaused all my resources and still had a desert to cross. Compression is an action similar to the instinctive drawing of blood away from the surface of the body in preparation for battle. It is appropriate in situations in which you must go on, and contracting, collapsing, expansion, all the other movements of your being, won't do. Then compression works, and works well. But if you get stuck there so that you can't let down and open up—can't release the clamp—the result is depression and discomfort. Of course, if you are crossing a great uncertain desert and have no other options, you are less concerned with feeling good than with simply continuing on to the other side. If, when you *get* to the oasis, you neither drop to the ground in relief nor throw your arms up and shout, then you can be sure you are stuck. Most of us know this response so intimately that we find it hard to recognise in ourselves; it is our deepest habit of distribution and we often find it difficult to see.

So let me put it another way: Compression is what happens when you won't let yourself down and you won't let yourself up—nor really in or out. You collect a lot of tightly bound, dense energy towards the middle of your body—often in the torso, from the pelvic floor to the neck, but not always. A person stuck in collapse often feels a kind of fatigued, drained-out depression, but a person stuck in compression feels a first-rate, grimey, gritty, guilt-ridden, intense and involuted depression. The feeling tone of this energy distribution is one of being trapped but capable: "I can take it." "This isn't so bad." When you are unconsciously exerting that "in-from-both-ends" kind of pressure, it's hard to let yourself feel good by allowing your energy to move. (It would hardly matter whether the movement was down or up, in or out; any energetic

41

movement would improve how you felt.) Once established, compression resists most of all the pulsation that would bring pleasure. What would spring open the trap is experienced as frightening.

The Breath of Life

Diffusion/condensation, expansion/contraction, and collapsing/ballooning are normal movements across a spectrum, much like breathing itself. Compression doesn't have an outbreath, so to speak. Or an inbreath. It's held between in and out, which is what makes it so uncomfortable. Containment is related to compression as yes is to no. Containment produces power and pleasure and reserves of energy. Unlike compression, it evolves from a flexible strength that allows pulsation of the field. It is the line between control and abandon. In the first of Carlos Casteneda's books about his encounter with Don Juan, the shaman talks about the Path of the Warrior. He says that the warrior walks the line between control and abandon. The balance between these two actions, in and of itself, creates flow. In any of the exercises we do here, we are learning to walk this line. We move into a position that requires control to maintain and, in that position, abandon ourselves to it, surrender to its effects. When we learn to manage these two things simultaneously, we produce a condition of containment. To describe what's involved is a bit difficult because it isn't often modelled for us as children. We learn repression and explosion of our energies instead.

EXERCISE 20: Consider that we have chosen a boundary (whether consciously or unconsciously) and, within that boundary, we have induced a condensation of the field so that the energy within the boundary is denser than the energy outside of it. Automatically, there will be a pressure to expand the boundary. First, allow the expansion and enjoy those good feelings. Your boundary will tend to expand until the densities inside and outside are equalised.

But suppose that you don't want to experience oneness through diffusion or to merge with another person in that particular way. Suppose instead that you want to maintain this particular condensation of energy and this boundary—you want to *contain* this particular pressure to expand. At the same time, you don't want to contract or compress the energy; you want it to be both flowing *and* dense. Think of it as having sufficient muscle tone in your energetic body to hold the boundary without compressing, without contracting, without expanding, without ballooning, without diffusing. The way to do this is to create or allow a pulsation, a "feathering" of your field at its boundary. Containment is characterised by this pulsation of the boundary.

If you look through a microscope at a happy, normally functioning one-celled creature, it will seem to shimmer. This visible shimmer arises from its pulsation. The pulsation is that cell "walking the line between control and abandon," a part of its self-containment within that membrane which is its physical boundary. It contains itself within the membrane *with* the membrane, and the membrane pulsates. A characteristic of the creature's being alive is that it pulsates. If its boundary membrane doesn't pulsate at all, the membrane loses flexibility, and a rigid cell is soon dead.

We are far more complex in structure, but we, too, are composed of boundaries made of membranes that pulse with life, that must pulsate in order to live: the heart sac, the lungs, the peristaltic intestines, all the billions of cell membranes, and the skin that marks the physical limit of the body. We can and must pulsate at any or all of these boundaries, yet it often frightens us to do so. Binding ourselves between yes and no, we are boundaries within boundaries within boundaries. In this exercise, we are practising the voluntary formation of an energetic boundary that contains our physical boundaries. We invite pulsation of that energetic boundary, which in turn invites pulsation of deeper and deeper inner boundaries—invitations to walk between control and abandon. (See Appendix B.)

Collect and condense enough energy to give yourself something to play with. (You can use the exercises from earlier in the chapter.) Choose a boundary that allows you to feel resilience in your field and the desire to expand. Allow the pressure to expand you a little bit, a few inches or a foot, and then bring your energy back in to the earlier point. Allow the expansion and the drawing back, over and over. Gradually, allow the expansion over a smaller and smaller range. Notice the sensations and feelings that arise. Be sure to allow yourself to make appropriate sounds.

When we are in harmony with ourselves and our environment—

from which we are *not* energetically separate, remember—such pulsation happens spontaneously. Practising pulsation helps us to re-establish in a conscious way the harmony most babies are born with and most adults have lost.

Pulsation is a characteristic of containment and is pleasurable to the organism. Containment and the surrender to pulsation are what make higher and higher levels of organismic charge possible. Developing and containing charge creates—*is*, in a way—excitement. This charge creates the dipole, the energetic "distance" and "push", that leads to the desire for union and the capacity for it.

All the feelings and sensations we experience, whether we identify them as emotions or not, arise from movement in the body (including the energy body). Feelings are rhythmic and pulsatory in origin, which means that all feelings can be pleasurable. I know this is a radical statement. We don't experience all feelings as pleasurable because we are taught to clamp down on some of them, usually because other people find them uncomfortable. Contract and compress—stop 'em at the neck, stop 'em at the tail. This creates a standing wave that is uncomfortable for *you*. If you are terrified and you run screaming from what threatens you, you will no longer name that energy "terror". If you will notice (as you run, of course), what you are experiencing is enormously pleasurable and satisfying. Again, if you are angry and move into action to change what needs changing, the energy loses the name of anger so long as you allow a relaxed, contained movement within yourself. Anger, fear, and sadness get labelled as "bad feelings" because of the effects of repressing energetic movement. Conversely, any wave of feeling can be made uncomfortable if you clamp down on it, including orgasm.

EXERCISE 21: Try that. At the moment of orgasm, contract or compress. Make no sounds. (Just don't write me a letter of complaint when I'm right about it.)

It's important to notice that I am talking here about energetic movement, not necessarily physical action. I'm not handing out a *carte blanche* for impulsive behaviour. I'm not suggesting that you hit people if you are angry or that you can run from everything that frightens you. I *am* saying that, whatever the situation, there are energetic alternatives to compression and contraction, energetic alternatives to hurting yourself and feeling bad about being. The keys to those alternatives are containment and pulsation. It's helpful, also, to keep away from making judgments about any of these energetic movements, even compression. They all serve positive purposes, even though you can also give yourself trouble with any of them.[8]

We are the collection of energy within a limited vessel. It is our grounding in physical existence, our bodily being, simultaneous with our capacity for energetic merger that permits the event we call orgasm. Energetically, you can set your own limits on the vessel, contain energy within it, and dissolve it at will. Without containment, energy doesn't collect properly. A person may be left with the frustrations of not collecting enough energy or of having nowhere to go with it, of having energy drift off or drain away, of never fully releasing outwards or inwards.

If you can imagine an Ideal Human Container—though, as with Boyle's Ideal Gas, there is no ideal—that ideal energetic container would be infinitely expandable, infinitely contractable, infinitely diffusable, infinitely condensable, with boundaries ranging from steel-like rigidity to mist-like permeability. The miracle is how nearly we have access to that range.

Notes

1. This is the only part of the book that I anticipate might be boring. If you find it so, please hold your nose and plow on; it's important.

2. "Too far" means losing our capacity to act appropriately and to release at need into expansion.

3. Though energetically they are saying "no" all the time.

4. "Too far" in this case means beyond what we can contain; see the later section on containment.

5. Or, perhaps, to become aware of the one-ness. Talking about energetic realities requires some shifts and some language we haven't made yet.

6. Sometimes people with diffuse fields eat a lot to give themselves an imitation of the protective "thickness" that greater density of field would provide them.

7. So far as I know—I'm a diffuser myself. Tony Richardson, M.D., Ph.D., suggests these disadvantages: isolation in relation to other beings, a sense of staleness, and inertia. He adds, "Overcondensed fields are very heavy to carry around." These disadvantages arise from lack of movement and pulsation.

8. Readers familiar with bioenergetics and the developmental character structures of Alexander Lowen will notice the following correlations: habitual contraction with schizoid character; habitual energetic collapse with oral character; habitual compression with masochistic character; habitual ballooning with psychopathy; habitual expansion (energetic pressure outwards) with rigid character. My own experience is that these energetic movements are characteristic responses to specific threatening situations and occur no matter the age at which the threat is experienced. Like other aspects of character structure, however, most *habits* of energetic response are established early. Changes in structure allow more energetic strength and flexibility; conversely, more energetic movement often catalyses changes in structure.

9
Getting Energy from Here to There

The life energy we are dealing with here has the quality of flow, just like electricity in a wire. Also like the electricity in a wire, it encounters resistance. The wire provides resistance because of its structure and also because of this structure provides a direction for the flow of electricity. A corroded wire prevents flow.

The resistance to flow we encounter in our bodies is partly the natural resistance of form to change (our tendency to stay the same shape, rather than become butterflies or tree sloths) and partly the resistance of experience. Some of our experiences teach us to contract against life—against ourselves to preserve ourselves, in fact—and this slows down the flow or even interrupts it. When this happens, our first step is to begin to re-establish the conditions for flow. From here on, there will be lots of exercises, much more doing than talking about doing.

EXERCISE 22: Stand in the basic position: feet parallel, weight over the centre of your feet, knees relaxed and slightly bent, pelvis relaxed and free, belly relaxed, shoulders relaxed and in balance, jaw relaxed, eyes relaxed. With eyes closed, feel for any sense of flow in your body. With your inner vision, look for any "breaks in the wire". Now lift your hands and reach up and back gently. Keeping your head upright, arch your back slightly. Visualise yourself as the "wire"—the energetic connection—between earth and sky. Feel again for a sense of flow. Stay with the sense of connectedness for as long as you are comfortable. Make a sound along the wire. Be aware of any feelings that arise (yearning, discomfort, confusion, anger, etc.). Expand the energy of the sensations you feel and allow them to move throughout your body (and beyond your body, if you like). Rest, sitting or lying down, for several minutes. Continue to allow the movement and expansion of energy.

This exercise invites a flow of energy through your body. As you allow yourself to become aware of the energy freed and arising in response to the exercise, notice the pattern of movement. Up, down, in, out, variations on all these. Is one movement easier for you than the others?

We can use the energy we have invited through this exercise to practise the basic means of moving energy. For many of us, the first step in moving energy is to get some available, that is, to raise our overall energy level. The most basic ways to free up more energy are breathing and movement.

Breath is important in moving energy because it supplies oxygen to the cells. The right amount of oxygen means that each cell burns a clean flame and produces more available energy.

EXERCISE 23: This energising breath, with the splendid name The Breath of Fire, comes from yoga. Breathe through your nose ten times as rapidly, deeply, and forcefully as you can; then breathe normally three times. Repeat twice.

All of these exercises are potent, so be respectful. If you have been practising a repressive or contractive breath for some time, a little bit of this may go a very long way. If you start to feel dizzy, pause in the exercise, sit or lie quietly, and be aware of the sensations and inner movements that arise in response to the breath. Allow them to expand throughout your body (and beyond, if you like). As we breathe, so we feel. There are calming breaths, happy breaths, passionate breaths, angry breaths, fearful breaths, sad breaths, repressive breaths, and energising breaths—in fact, a different and characteristic breathing pattern for every way you feel. You may suppose that we breathe in these characteristic ways *because* of what we are feeling. As Namgyal Rinpoche says, "Every time you experience an emotional change, the breathing pattern changes."[1] The reverse, however, is also true—that if we breathe in the way characteristic of a certain feeling, we will begin to feel that feeling.

Movement also can be used to get access to "static" energy. All exercise that you love does this. Movement to create or free energy is always intimately associated with the response of your breath to the movement, so . . . as you move, breathe. Let the breath follow the movement.

EXERCISE 24: Try this old exercise from the Sufi tradition. Hands over your head, jump vigorously up and down, thumping your heels on the floor and hollering HOO! HOO! HOO!

as loudly as you can.

Be respectful: stop before you fall down. Sit or lie quietly.

This is very noticeably a movement exercise. You will see that it also has a profound effect on breathing. What other effects do you notice? In doing the exercise, be respectful of your current limits. Be aware of what suits you: ten seconds, 30 seconds, several minutes. Be aware of the sensations moving in your being. As before, allow them to expand. Fuse your consciousness with the energy moving in you. Let the energy move you into walking or dancing around the room.

In this exercise, we move the whole body. Movement in any *part* of the body focusses energy in that part and, in addition, allows energy to arise from the tissues in the area. We can also use movement in one part of the body to offer energy to another part. Friction is the most obvious form of this kind of movement. In Chapter 6, we experimented with rubbing our hands together to charge them. That energy in the hands can then be donated to any other part of the body—or to someone else. We also use friction as a way to move energy into the genitals in the more usual kinds of masturbation and foreplay. Friction is not, however, the only way to use movement in directing energy into the genitals.

EXERCISE 25: For pelvic breathing, stand in basic position. Use your hands to outline the bone structure of your pelvis (see illustration). Notice it is the only bowl-shape in the body. Visualise it as your reserve cup of energy. Now, bending your knees a bit more, let your pelvis begin to move with your breath. As you breathe in, the top of your pelvis tips forward and your rear moves back. The bend is at the sacro-lumbar joint, *not* in your middle back. Be gentle, not forcing. As you exhale, the top of your pelvis moves back and the pubic bone lifts forward and slightly up. Let the movement follow the breath. Join your consciousness with the movement in your pelvis. Feel into the flavour of the energy arising from the movement, whatever it may be: gentle, powerful, angry, seeking, desirous, and so forth. Let the movement express that flavour. Make a sound that is also expressive of the feeling. Notice that the flavour may change. Experiment with various qualities and rhythms of

49

(a) Pelvis cocked   (b) Aligned position
backward

Movement of the Pelvis
(Drawn, after Gorman, by Judith Santry.)

(a) Pelvis cocked backward   (b) Aligned position

In pelvic breathing, the pelvis moves further forward (up and through) on
the outbreath.

movement, and see if the feeling you sense changes with the movement. Continue as long as you are comfortable or feel pleasure in the experience. Sit or lie quietly, allowing expansion of the feelings and sensations within you.

You can use this exercise
• to increase energy in your pelvis
• to release energy held static in your pelvis
• to intensify sensation in the merging and separating exercise (see pages 65–66)
• to increase awareness of your pelvis and genitals
• to increase confidence in your sexuality.
Pelvic breathing can be added to many exercises to vary and intensify their effects for grounding, charging, centering, and focusing. Try the following variation.

EXERCISE 26: Lie on your back on a comfortable surface. Bend your knees and put your feet on the ground about a hand's length from your buttocks. (This is called "grounding your feet".) In this position, breathe pelvically. Again, allow your awareness to merge with the movement, and notice what feelings arise. Allow the movement to be expressive. Join sound to the movement. You are a conduit; allow life to flow in you (guiltlessly, to the extent that you *can* now). Vary what you experience by reaching softly upwards with your arms or by allowing them to rest gently open and outstretched on the ground.

Support the sensation of flow where you experience it. Avoid judgment. Make no comparisons. What you are experiencing now is what you can experience. If you experience a little sensation or movement or flow or vibration, let it be enough; embrace it; it will open you to more. If you feel only the frustration of no movement, no flow, then rest in the recognition that the frustration is that energy moving towards movement. Embrace the intention, and relax. On the other hand, if you feel the experience becoming too intense, be patient; roll gently over on to your left side and rest there, allowing the sensations you feel to expand and diffuse, letting go of intensity.

Notice that pelvic breathing combines breath and movement to direct energy into a specific area. It is very important in doing any of these exercises to participate in them with full awareness, to *become* the movement and the breath. In my youth, the tendency was to do your thirty jumping jacks on automatic pilot. Here I am urging you to let your awareness enter into the event. As you experience the effect of the movement and breath, express it in sound. As you express it in sound, you will alter or intensify what you are experiencing. (This is genuine biofeedback.) Such sounds with movement may catalyse deep feelings. Respect your feelings and respect your limits.

EXERCISE 27—HOW TO RECOGNISE YOUR LIMITS: If, as you are doing an exercise, you find you are *breathing less or tightening up* in some part of your body *in order to go on* with the exercise, then you have exceeded your current limits. Learn to recognise that this is *about* to happen. Stop then. Rest in the experience at that point when you can remain relaxed. That resting may stretch your limits so that you can go on a bit further. It *may*; be conservative. You want to be able to repeat these experiments. Pushing on and on without respect for your current organismic limits may create a backlash such that you never want to hear the word "pelvis" again.

These last exercises direct energy specifically into the pelvis. Later I will introduce you to exercises that support the spontaneous redistribution of that energy (see "But I Can't . . . " and "The Lover Within"). The pelvis, however, is not the genitals (though it includes them), and that creates confusion. It is possible to move quite a lot of energy into your pelvis and still have "interruptions" in the energy connections between pelvis and genitals. So you may find that charging your pelvis with such exercises leaves you still with a vagueness or frustration in your genitals, rather than excitement. If so, or if you want to increase the clarity and intensity of focus there, take a look at Dr. Kegel's exercises invented to help women with urinary incontinence after pregnancy. Shyly, they began to report to him improvements in their sex lives.

Kegel's exercises involve rhythmic contraction and release (i.e., pulsation) of the pubococcygeal muscles of the perineum (see illustrations). These are the muscles we use to control the perineal sphincters. They also pulse rhythmically during orgasm. There was some puzzlement as to why doing Kegel exercises would increase orgasmic responsiveness, and suggestions were made that, somehow, increased tone in these muscles increased proprioception in the vaginal wall.[2] This is likely to be so; increased tonus increases awareness in any area. It is also true that increasing the attention or consciousness directed to an area increases circulation and tonus in the musculature there.[3] Look at the illustration, and notice that movement of these muscles also causes the hood of the clitoris to slide up and down, revealing and concealing that sensitive organ. Don't forget that such friction is also a way of directing energy into a specific area (see the hand rubbing exercise, pages 21–22).

Whatever else Kegels may do, they are a *charging* exercise without equal for the genitals. They bring increased energy, attention, intention, oxygen, tone, circulation, and *pulsation* to the genital tissues—for men as well as women. Like all the exercises here, Kegels must be done with awareness and full participation. If you bore yourself and make them mechanical, the tissues will not enliven, no matter how many times you prime the pump.

EXERCISE 28: Familiarise yourself with the muscles in question. Look at the illustrations of male and female perineal muscles. Focus your awareness on and in the muscles you use to regulate the flow of urine. Try it in the bathroom, playfully. Later your awareness will become much more specific. When you've located the muscles, begin to pulse them in and out, a rhythmic contraction and release. Experiment with different rhythms. If you are female, you may notice a specific sensation of the hood sliding over your clitoris. Pulsation of the perineal muscles encourages engorgement of clitoris and vaginal walls. If you are male, notice that these are the muscles that "flip" your penis in excitement. They directly influence tumescence. (Kalahari bushmen strengthen these muscles until they can draw their testicles up inside the body for protection during the hunt.) Try a variety of movement patterns; there are many muscles involved. Try the effects of lying down, sitting, and walking as you do the exercise. Let your breath stay free to respond. As always, enter into the sensations that arise with the movements. Express the sensations in sound. You may find your pelvis wants to join in to reinforce the charge and sensation. (As you surrender to the sensa-

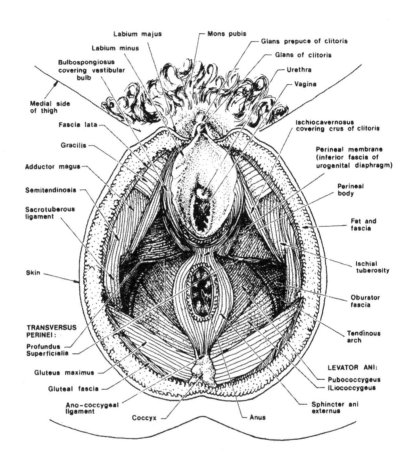

Labium majus
Labium minus
Bulbospongiosus
covering vestibular
bulb
Medial side
of thigh
Fascia lata
Gracilis
Adductor magus
Semitendinosis
Sacrotuberous
ligament
Skin
TRANSVERSUS
PERINEI:
Profundus
Superficialis
Gluteus maximus
Gluteal fascia
Ano-coccygeal
ligament

Mons pubis
Glans prepuce of clitoris
Glans of clitoris
Urethra
Vagina
Ischiocavernosus
covering crus of clitoris
Perineal membrane
(inferior fascia of
urogenital diaphragm)
Perineal
body
Fat and
fascia
Ischial
tuberosity
Oburator
fascia
Tendinous
arch
LEVATOR ANI:
Pubococcygeus
iliococcygeus
Sphincter ani
externus

Coccyx
Anus

Superficial Muscles of the Female Perineum
(Drawn, after Gorman, by Judith Santry.)

54

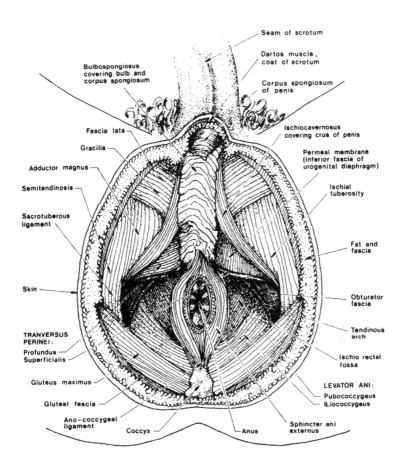

Seam of scrotum

Dartos muscle,
coat of scrotum

Bulbospongiosus
covering bulb and
corpus spongiosum

Corpus spongiosum
of penis

Ischiocavernosus
covering crus of penis

Fascia lata

Gracilis

Perineal membrane
(inferior fascia of
urogenital diaphragm)

Adductor magnus

Semitendinosis

Ischial
tuberosity

Sacrotuberous
ligament

Fat and
fascia

Skin

Obturator
fascia

Tendinous
arch

TRANVERSUS
PERINEI:
Profundus
Superficialis

Ischio rectal
fossa

Gluteus maximus

LEVATOR ANI:
Pubococcygeus
ILiococcygeus

Gluteal fascia

Ano-coccygeal
ligament

Coccyx

Anus

Sphincter ani
externus

Superficial Muscles of the Male Perineum
(Drawn, after Gorman, by Judith Santry.)

55

tions released by this movement, you may experience a spontaneous release of energy somewhere in your body. Allow that to lead you into a deeper surrender.) Continue with the exercise as long as you feel pleasure or until you get tired. As the muscles tire, be glad they're getting stronger.

Pause now and consider what we've been doing: breathing and moving. This breathing and moving has been in response to an *intention* to breathe and to move. Intentionality in the muscles is immediate in response to thought. Simultaneous. If you can conceive the action, the body is *in that moment* prepared to act. All that separates thought and action is consent. Visualise intention fanning out through the whole body and activating the entire array of synapses. A consensus among the relevant synapses give "consent" to the action.*

In practical terms, this means that we can move very quickly when we need to—with intention, but without conscious "thought". It also means that, if we have old messages in the synaptic network chanting "Hell, no, we won't go" or "Momma wouldn't like that", we may have to negotiate consent, give ourselves new neurological permissions.

There is something else implied that may sound a bit fantastical: this power of intention can move energy without any other "action" on our part. Usually we will want the assistance of breath and movement and other methods to empower our intention, but it is possible simply to intend a movement of energy. The energy will move as intended. It may only happen in dribbles at first, but with practise it will get easier and stronger.

Visualisation is a great tool for "boosting" intention. You may have read about athletes improving their performance by visualising themselves play superbly. Try this old acting exercise (an easier version of Exercise 14).

EXERCISE 29: Pick a room you like. Not too big, not too small. Stand in it, look it over, feel the size of it. Now fill it with yourself, with your energy.

In acting terms, this is called "taking the stage". In our terms, it is called "expanding the energy body to the boundaries of the room". You can fill it, knowing that you are *literally* altering the energetic character of yourself in the room. Or you can "imagine" or "pretend" that you are filling it. This will have exactly the same effect, if perhaps not so powerfully at first. Your energy will follow your intention even in imagination; you will fill the room simply by pretending that you are doing so. The more strongly you intend it, the more vividly you imagine it, the more densely you will fill it and the more charged the energy will be.

This exercise uses intention and direction. You intend to fill the room and, by intending it, you direct your energy into the room. The skills of placing your energy where you want it make it possible to move out of old "stuck" patterns. Sexually, you can have energy "stuck" away from your genitals, as if your sexuality were a fire zone to be abandoned; or you can have energy stuck *in* your genitals and spend a lot of time in unnecessary and uncreative frustration.

We can use these tools (intention, visualisation, direction, breath, and movement) to build energy pathways into parts of the body where there is an interruption of flow—whether interrupted because we are blocked by old experience or simply because we are entering new territory altogether. The building of such pathways is common in training for martial arts and in certain Buddhist meditations.

EXERCISE 30: Stand in the basic position. First, visualise a point of light or centre of power about four fingers breadth down from your navel. You may already be familiar with this centre; if not, visualising it will help strengthen both the centre and your awareness of it. Bend your knees slightly and relax them (*inside* the knee) to facilitate flow of energy; you may feel some vibration in your legs. Allow whatever sensations of vibration and flow you experience (within the limits of comfort). Now visualise channels about one inch in diameter running from this centre in the pelvis out and down through your legs, through the centre of your feet, and into the ground. Intend flow from the centre through these channels; direct it. You can reinforce and strengthen your intention by any one or more of the following:
• Breathe pelvically.
• Visualise a channel through your throat down to the

pelvic centre. Let the inhaled breath "feed" energy into the centre. On the exhalation, let energy flow as before down the channels into the ground.

- Lift one leg and slowly, powerfully, extend it on the exhalation, visualising the flow of energy through the channel. Repeat with other leg.
- On the exhalation make a long, strong, focussed "ocean" sound through your mouth as you visualise the flow. (This greatly strengthens the "direction" of the flow and is similar to a *ki-ai* in martial arts, though not explosive.)

Try these one at a time before you put them together.

EXERCISE 31: Try this similar experiment with your arms and hands. Visualise an energy centre in the middle of your chest and channels running from this heart centre through your arms and out through the centres of your palms. Begin by moving energy through these channels by simple intention and direction. Then reinforce these by

- matching breath to visualisation
- extending your arms on the exhalation
- making a sound on the exhalation.

EXERCISE 32: In aikido, energy flow is focussed and directed through the side of the hand like a blade, and the flow is intended from the pelvic centre rather than the heart, but the procedure is otherwise the same. Try this variation, and notice any differences in feeling and sensation of the energy passing through your arms and hands as it comes from the heart and as it comes from the pelvic centre (*hara*).

In these exercises, you have been introduced to all the basic skills you need to practise voluntary energy distribution. Choose one or two and do them regularly for three or four months. During that time, don't concern yourself with how "well" you are doing; just prepare the ground and water the seeds. If you let yourself continue to do the exercises with attention but without concern about the results, opening will begin. Pathways have to be built for the energy to move through and past the arbitrary boundaries you have built, as well as into entirely new territories of experience. You can go deeper and deeper. First, energy flows "around" the body; the tissues of the body do not feel deeply touched. Later the energy flows through the body, as if along the interstices of the cells.

Finally, the substance of the cells themselves begin to pulsate.[5] Give yourself time, and offer the process respect, playfulness, practice.

Notes

1. Namgyal Rinpoche, *Body, Speech, and Mind*, p. 112.

2. Did anyone ever ask what happened for men when they did Kegel exercises?

3. Gerda Alexander, teaching workshop, Berkeley, March 1984.

4. This approach to intentionality reflects the teachings of anatomist David Gorman.

5. See Appendix B for a fuller description of this developmental sequence.

10
Union and Separation

If you aren't yet confused about what love is, you ought to be. It isn't just that we love our parents, we love our mates, we love kittens and apple pie, we love hang-gliding, we love potato chips, we love . . .

No, it isn't just that we spray the word around as if it meant everything and nothing. Most of us are desperately hungry for *something*, almost undefined, that will make life bearable. Some of us are so hungry that we deny there is anything to be hungry for. Most often we march—or drift—grimly through life, waiting. When we meet someone or something that promises to satisfy that hunger, we surge towards it/him/her. Or withdraw, stroking our despair. Now is this "love"? We call it love, and it certainly is desire; but how often it turns out to be greed, faintly disguised. *Can* we be loving as long as we are so desperately hungry?

We are inclined to think of union and separation as happening *between* people, though of course we also feel in union with ourselves or cut off from ourselves, united with our community or not, in harmony with life or not. And it's not that union is good and separation is bad. As with other movements of energy, each has its advantages and disadvantages, and full functioning lies in the capacity for choice and a continuing balance and re-balance between the two.

Before we can truly unite with another, before we can be truly separate, we need to unite within ourselves. This need is not always clear to us. So it happens that one of the feelings that people most often feel is yearning. What we attach our yearning to depends on where we hold our energy in stasis and where, consequently, we hope for salvation—chest, groin, belly, head. What are you sure is going to fix things for you if only you can get it? Money, sex, power, love, god, unlimited chocolate chip cookies?

We can lose our self-union in many ways as we're growing up. Life[1] may be too frightening to stand, and so we lose our feet. Life may be too depriving to stand up to, and so we lose our backbone. Life may reject our fullness, and so we split heart from groin and lose our sexual unity. This sexual disunity within us leads us both to distrust the other we want for partner and to hope against hope for some salvation through him or her.

EXERCISE 33: Lie on your back with your feet grounded. Close your eyes and look inward. Where are you more at home—in your heart or in your groin? Does the power in your groin protect your heart or ignore it? Does your heart offer tenderness and generosity to your passion or pretend it doesn't exist? Bring heart and groin into your awareness simultaneously. What feelings and sensations arise? How do you feel about what you feel?

Close your eyes for a moment and be young; then open your eyes and remember those feelings as you read. Back when we are first beginning to experience ourselves as a separate energy pulsation—which is really how it is, if we manage to achieve that much—we begin to feel a longing for union. We have been in union and we have wanted separation, and we get separation and feel a longing for union. It isn't a terrible thing, this paradox; it's a wonderful thing. It's life beginning to know itself and reaching out to embrace itself. It's a natural and miraculous process. All kinds of creatures do it. Only we're about five years old, and we're reaching out with love, reaching out for union with all the power of our being, from groin and heart. It's not yet in a grown-up form, but the feeling is very powerful, intense, and potent. We reach out, usually to the opposite sex parent, to the other pole of union, the opposite. Because of the strength of the feelings, because they are full of pleasure and longing, and because they almost always touch on the heartbreak[2] that the parent has experienced, that opposite sex parent gets frightened and pulls back energetically, away from union. We almost always receive this as the heartbreaking news that our longing for union is not acceptable, that we must be less than whole, less than we are, or we will not be received.

I don't know how things would go if this message were received in another culture, but in our culture most of us are taught to split ourselves in two and to choose heart or groin. This is not an easy thing to do, but we manage it, mostly by contraction of the diaphragm—the big muscle that in fact divides the body in two.

In the general way of things, men are encouraged to and do choose their groins. There is a lot of pressure on them to do that and to abandon their hearts. Women, because there is a lot of pressure on them to do so, often choose their hearts; they remember how to be gentle and nurturing and enfolding and giving, but they abandon their groins. Not everybody cuts in two completely, thank God; there's some communication back and forth. But many times a man looks for a woman who offers him a heart and, however temporarily, access to his tender feelings; and a woman looks for a man who offers her, however temporarily, the power of desire and generation. Self-union is about getting that "other" back within us.

We feel longing for union: with another, within ourselves, ultimately with all that is. The more powerful the desire for union, the more of life it takes to satisfy it. So you might pause and hold on to a little compassion for your partner, who's being asked to stand in for life. When these feelings are catalysed, we demand—with a complete lack of common sense—that our partner be *all* to us, giving all and receiving all. That union between two grown-ups, or two people who are in the process of becoming grown-ups, can be a remarkably intense thing. It touches on much more than, "Do you love me?". It touches on, "How can I take life into myself?" and "How can I be whole and offer myself wholly to being?". It's a deep place. When you love someone, and you desire full union and your partner fears it, it can be very frustrating for both of you. Recognise the probability that if your partner were suddenly fully willing, you would discover your own fear. Deep union can be very frightening. We are drawn towards it like an abyss and pull back from the edge, again and again. The pleasure of it is so intense that it's possible to feel that you are going to dissolve, melt, lose yourself altogether and forever. A loving passion of this kind is transformative and almost irresistible.

EXERCISE 34: Lie on your back, comfortably, with your feet grounded. Laugh for five minutes. Accept no excuses. Laugh. Ho ho ho. Ha ha. Hee. Laugh.

EXERCISE 35: Lie on your back on a comfortable firm surface, feet grounded. Place a small cushion under your chest. Let your arms be gently open and outstretched to the side. Breathe pelvically. Feel the sensations in your pelvis. Merge with them. Continue to breathe pelvically, and slowly raise your arms as if to embrace your beloved. Let the lifting of your arms be slow enough that you can feel each moment of movement. You may feel trembling or vibration in your arms and legs. Feel free to make sound throughout. Let heart and groin remember each other. Visualise an energy channel connecting the two. Allow heart feeling to touch pelvis and groin. How does that effect the movement of your pelvis? What is the message? Allow energy from your pelvis and groin to flow upwards to your chest and heart. What feelings and sensations arise? Which is easier? Is either one scary? What do heart and groin say, speaking together? (Go slowly; respect your limits.)

One of the things you need to decide is whether you really want to risk re-encountering your power and your vulnerability. I think it's worth it, but I also know what it was like to get here. With these exercises, we begin to touch on feelings that most people take care all their lives never to feel more than once: anguish, heartbreak,[2] powerlessness, as well as union, ecstasy, and bliss. This is another issue of wholeness and self-union. Some people separate power from vulnerability and will not let themselves be touched. Others cherish their vulnerability because it allows them to be touched, but stagger back from their own power. You can't go deeply into the experience of pleasure if you cut yourself off from either the tiger or the flower.

I remember vividly the morning I woke up knowing there was a difference between the capacity to be touched and *expecting* to be hurt. All my life up to that time, whenever I opened myself, I was expecting to be hurt. If you open yourself to both the vulnerability that allows you to be touched and the power that gives passion and protection, life is your lover.

EXERCISE 36: Charge your hands by rubbing them together. Feel the energy in your hands and between them. Experience it as your life and your presence. With your hands, bring that energy towards your heart. When do you feel touched?

EXERCISE 37: Repeat Exercise 36 while breathing pelvically.

EXERCISE 38: Repeat the exercise, while breathing pelvically and facing a partner. Let your hands approach those of your partner. What do you feel? Let your hands move gently toward your partner's heart as his hands move toward your heart. When do you touch him? When are you touched? Be respectful of your feelings and of his. Allow the sensations and feelings that arise to move and expand throughout your body (and beyond if you like). If you need to move away from your partner, respect that need. If the two of you wish to embrace, do so.

Doing these exercises can prime your feelings of longing. As you charge your hands and bring that energy to your heart, the energy will want to move out into your arms again. This may catalyse longing. What do you do with your longing? Can you feel it in the tissues of your body? We are often taught not to reach out with longing and power. It's frightening because we remember rejection and our loss of wholeness. We tend to limit the number of people we're willing to reach towards (even a little), the number of situations in which we are willing to let our energy flow out and contact another person. We fear both the power and the vulnerability of our longing. So it often happens that we experience the desire to reach out *and* a contraction away from reaching at the same moment. Those two things happening together can create a pain, a literal pain in the chest. A person who has in the past reached from the whole of her being towards another person and been denied will often experience revivification of her heart space as pain. She may feel that she is dying, having a heart attack. It is a deep anguish. That's why I ask you again and again to be kind and loving to yourself in the exercises, to avoid judgment, make no comparisons, and respect your current limits. We're all in this together. The question of how willing we are to touch and be touched may never be fully answered. It seems we can always go deeper into life, touch more deeply, be more deeply touched. Show less and less resistance in the wire.

The movement towards self-union prepares for union with the other. Union with self and other prepares for union with life. Self-union also allows energetic separation from the other that is not withdrawal, not rejection.

EXERCISE 39: Stand facing a partner. Negotiate the distance between you. Pick a distance at which you both feel separate.[3] Close your eyes. Feel the bones of your spine and your spine as a whole as distinctly as you can; notice (without judgment) any bits you can't yet feel. Visualise your energy gathering together and forming a supportive column centred on your spine and continuing to the ground. Notice the sensations associated with this energy distribution. Are they familiar? Is it easy? Do you like it? When you have your energy collected in this way and fairly stable (no judgments), open your eyes and look at your partner. Notice what happens. If your energy flows out towards your partner, let that happen. Then close your eyes and draw your energy back into a column centred around your spine. (If your energy does *not* automatically flow out towards your partner, intend that, visualise it, and release your energy towards merger. Then draw it back into a column.) When you are ready, once again open your eyes. This time, see if you can hold the column in place for a few seconds before releasing your energy to merge with the other. Enjoy merging. Close your eyes, and re-form the column. Repeat the separation-merger-separation process several times. Notice that it gets easier. It will also probably get more powerful. (This is a charging exercise for couples in addition to its other virtues.) Then open your eyes, hold the separation, enjoy the sensations. Release into merger; enjoy the sensations. Allow yourself sound. Then, *eyes open* and contactful, draw your energy back into a column supporting your spine. Enjoy the sensations of being separate but present. Enjoy the charge between you and your partner. Then, if you like, release into merger and embrace your partner. Notice your preferences. Which is easier—to be separate or merged? Which is more pleasurable? When? Safer? When?

EXERCISE 40: Repeat the basic merging and separation process, this time breathing pelvically as you stand first with your eyes closed and then looking at your partner. If you feel comfortable, and the impulse is there, you may also want to reach out with your arms towards your partner. Try it with your eyes closed and then with them open. Continue to merge and separate energetically (as long as you are comfortable) in order to strengthen these energetic "muscles" under conditions of higher charge. Allow yourself to be aware of the feelings and sensations that arise. Allow them to move and expand through you (and towards and through your partner if you like). Expressive sound will stretch you energetically and intensify what is happening. After the exercise, let your partner know how you feel.

EXERCISE 41: With pelvic breathing and eye contact, gradually let your arms reach out to the side and forward (making a bowl shape). Slowly let your fingertips touch those of your partner. Continue pelvic breathing and allow your fingertips to pulse towards and away on the breath. Allow expressive sounds.

Often it happens in relationships (and within ourselves) that an imbalance arises between giving and taking. The following exercise helps to bring these two aspects of flow back into harmony.

EXERCISE 42: Sitting or lying comfortably, become aware of your breath. Be aware without judgment. Allow yourself to know what you want for yourself. Be specific. Pick one thing, and breathe it in. Let yourself know of something you want to give. Breathe it out into the universe. Continue until your imagination or your courage fails you. Notice your resistance to giving . . . or to taking. Notice your fears at even *imagining* this giving and taking. Notice the sensations that arise and allow them to expand. Remember that every tightness, every holding back, is a gift of life waiting to be unwrapped.

There are many exercises that support union *and* separation, power *and* vulnerability, giving *and* taking. Shortly you'll begin to make up your own.

When you get to be a grown-up, and you're out on the edges of what people know how to do, you blaze a trail—inside, with yourself, and outside, with other people. Don't forget the life that isn't people. You may find it easier to practice with a tree. Flowers and cats and puppies and geese and sea anemones. Cars, even. Stars.

One problem is that we get brought up on this hand-in-hand-happily-into-the-sunset routine, as if we are going to unite with *a* person (if we're *lucky*), and that's it, leaving out everything else in life. People are the only creatures who make any difficulty about it.

All the rest of creation is out there merging and separating, coming into being and dissolving, constantly, but without awareness. To do it with awareness is our gift. And our agony, often.

In the cultural metaphors we live by, mind lives in the head, love lives in the heart, desire lives in the groin. Some things we need not fight. We don't, however, have to limit ourselves to these metaphors. We don't have to live by limited definitions. If love lives in the heart, desire in the groin, and mind in the head, let awareness be at home everywhere.

Notes

1. I would like to emphasise that the experience of life we base such decisions on is not all of life, but we tend to act as if it were.

2. Heartbreak is a "technical" term referring to the anguish that arises when the desire for union is thwarted.

3. Usually this is not so very difficult to do. However, once a couple had to go outside on the sidewalk and back up 60 feet from each other in order to feel separate.

11

The Energetic Embrace

As I've said more than once, we get brought up with a lot of assumptions about things, especially about sex. Men are anatomically designed to penetrate and to be enfolded; women, to enfold and to be penetrated. However, the assumptions that have been hung on this anatomy are unnecessarily limiting.

Energy is not limited in these ways. Whether you are male or female, gay or straight, what you do with your energy is not limited by gender or anatomy.

As two people embrace, many movements of energy take place. The more choice you have in the movement of your energy, the more subtlety and variety you can bring to your union. As you move into embace, you can move your energy actively or passively; you can more your energy to penetrate or to enfold. Despite the current cultural assumptions, active energetic movement is not necessarily penetrative; neither is passive movement of energy necessarily enfolding. The four basic movements make a 2 x 2 matrix of possibilities for each person in the embrace. This is the matrix of embrace:

	ACTIVE	PASSIVE
PENETRATIVE	Most "heroes", the "normal" man, rapists: Gilgamesh John Wayne Lancelot	Young dying god: Attis James Dean Galahad
ENFOLDING	Great Mother: maternal to engulfing to devouring: Cybele Tiamat Medea Joan Crawford Isis Sorceress, witch: Circe Morgan le Fey Hecate	"Normal" women: Psyche Guenivere Penelope Merle Oberon Olivia de Haviland

In the spaces of the matrix, I've entered some of the judgments, opinions, assumptions, and expectations that "fit" the boxes. They are not all consistent. Which of them do you think are "true" or "false"? Jot down your own judgments as you become aware of them. Which of them can you let yourself be free of? At the same time, as you do the following exercise,[1] allow yourself to be aware of your preferences.

EXERCISE 43: Stand facing your partner at a comfortable distance. Decide between you who will first be active and who, passive. If you are to be active first, pause to collect yourself, feel your separateness, then look at your partner and actively send your energy out to enfold and surround him. (Your partner will at the same time passively penetrate you.) Without talking, note and enjoy the sensations of this experience. Make expressive sounds, if you like. Now draw your energy back. Collect it around your spine, as in the basic merging and separating exercise. Pause, again make eye contact with your partner, and again send your energy out actively, this time to penetrate his body energetically. (Your partner will simultaneously enfold you passively.) Be aware of your response. Let sound support and enlarge what you feel. Allow your experience to expand. Take your time. When you are ready, draw your energy back. Pause for awareness.

Now change places in the matrix, so that you now are moving your energy passively. As your partner actively enfolds you, allow your energy passively to penetrate him; let yourself be drawn in. Notice what sensations arise in each exchange and how you feel about them. Sound your feelings. When you are both ready, separate your energies. Pause. Then, as your partner actively penetrates you, feel the simultaneous sensations of passively enfolding him. Allow your feelings to expand throughout your body. Go as deeply into each aspect of the embrace as you feel comfortable doing. Allow yourselves to embrace physically if you both want to.

Draw your energy back. Each of you acknowledge your separateness and presence to the other. Sit together and talk about your experience. Be sure to notice which of these energetic movements you have opinions about. Which is easiest? Most pleasurable? Most comfortable? Most exciting? Do you feel uneasy with any of them? Does any one of them feel somehow "wrong"? Does your cultural training hint to you that only men—or only women—should do one or another of these movements? See if you are willing to let yourself enjoy all your energetic options in this embrace. Acknowledge your preferences without judgment.

Try this exercise with a number of people, though not necessarily one right after the other. Be aware of how the experience of embrace changes for you with each new partner. Do your preferences change?

Any of the exercises for pairs can be enjoyed as an embrace. Exercises for individuals can also be adapted for couples and can include embrace.

EXERCISE 44: Sit on the floor facing a partner with your knees open and the soles of your feet together. Move towards each other until you can sandwich your feet together lightly, i.e., your partner's feet embrace one of your feet, and your feet do the same for one of hers. Take time to notice the quality of the energetic contact. Allow the sensations you experience to expand through your whole body. Made a sound that resonates with what you experience. Consider allowing the energy of your sensations to flow out beyond you and into your partner.

Lean forward, each of you, and comfortably put your hands on your partner's shoulders. Again, take time to savour the contact and allow the sensations you feel to expand throughout your body and, perhaps, beyond you to your partner. You may notice that, with a partner you trust, you begin to form a circuit—that what you experience and allow to expand flows through her and returns to you flavoured by what she experiences. To deepen the connection and strengthen the circuit, lean together and gently touch foreheads. Make sounds that express what you feel. Try humming as well. While in this position, you can again try the varied energy exchanges of the matrix of embrace.

If you wish to go deeper into this exercise, you can now

begin a gentle circular movement from your hip joints. Stay energetically connected with your partner. Relax into the rhythm of the movement. Hum. Allow the movement to expand and to open your pelvis gently. Allow the circle to widen gradually. Be aware of the sensations that arise. Sound the feelings and allow them to expand through your whole being. Allow them to touch your partner. Rest together.

With your feet still overlapped with those of your partner, lie back and rest easy with your knees open to the sides. Relax the muscles of your legs as completely as possible; you might think of this as "freeing the bone".[2] Very, very slowly, lift your knees. Allow whatever vibration or trembling occurs. Rest for a time in each position where vibration occurs. Rest your attention in the vibration. Let the pulse of the vibration move down through your legs to your partner and up through your torso. Keep in mind that this is not an all-or-nothing process. Respect and encourage what you do experience rather than insisting on more. Make sounds. Hum. Do you notice any increase in vibration when your legs are at the same angle as your partner's? Gradually let your knees bring your legs up; then lower them again very slowly. Begin to lift them again. This time, feel within yourself for the position of most openness and flow in this spectrum of movement. Rest there. Again allow the energy of vibration to move up and down through your body. Allow the sensations you feel to expand and to express themselves in sound.

At any point in this exercise, should you feel you have taken on enough energy to stretch you, lie for several minutes on your left side or in some other comfortable position. You may choose to remain in contact physically with your partner or to be separate. (Remember that physical separation is not energetic separation and that energetic separation does not require rejection or emotional withdrawal.) In this resting time, you are allowing the energy you have released to stretch and expand you; you also allow time for the body literally to incorporate what you have learned. This resting phase of this exercise (and all the others) is just as important to the effect of the exercise as the active part. After you have rested, you and your partner may benefit from taking time to share in words something of what you have experienced.

EXERCISE 45: Sit with your partner in the position called by tantricas Yab-Yum. This means that the two of you sit front touching front with your legs scissored around each other and your arms supporting the embrace. It can include physical penetration or not; try it first without. (The illustration on page 75 shows a tantric couple embracing physically and energetically in Yab-Yum. This is what is referred to in the quotation in Chapter 1, "The Vajra of the Yab joined the Lotus of the Yum, and together they entered a state of great equanimity.") Breathe pelvically together. Try matching inhalation to inhalation and exhalation to exhalation at first so that your pelvises move apart on the inhalation and come together on exhalation. Move gently, and explore this contact. Experiment with various rhythms. Allow sound and the expansion of sensation. If you like, touch foreheads to complete the energetic circuit. To go deeper, try closing your eyes and lightly covering your partner's ears with your hands. (Check to make sure your shoulders are relaxed.) Go fully into the sensations that arise. As always, respect your limits; rest when you need to.

Vary the breathing pattern so that inhalation matches exhalation and your pelvises stay in contact as you breathe. Become one with the sensations that arise. Does this pattern feel different to you? How? Do you have a preference? Does your partner?

EXERCISE 46: Sit comfortably facing a partner. Each of you rub your hands together until they are warm and you can feel charge between them. Then slowly bring your index finger close to your partner's. Notice when you feel contact, when you feel touched. Stay at that distance a short while, allowing the charge to grow; bounce the field, if you like, by letting the two fingers approach a bit and withdraw a bit, over and over. Then bring your fingertips together. Close your eyes. While maintaining a sense of energetic contact, begin to move gently—a kind of dance of your arms and hands. Let your attention be on the sensations of flow and contact. Who is leading? Is anyone? Allow the movement to

Yab Yum
(Padmasambhava and Yeshe Tsogyel in physical
and energetic union. Detail drawn by Judith Santry from a scroll fresco
completed in 1980 by Lama Gonpo Rinpoche.)

expand and lead you to your feet if the flow invites it. Expand and contract the dance as it will, let it lift up and down. Rest. Be aware of your feelings and other responses to this temporary energetic marriage. Do you like it? Is it unnerving? Comforting? Exciting?[3] Often people find that this exercise gives them insight into their feelings and responses about union—the possibility of it, the frustration of it, and so on.

This chapter wouldn't be complete, as life is not, without looking at some of the common discomforts people experience as they move towards embrace and miss.

EXERCISE 47: With a partner you trust, stand facing each other at a comfortable distance and prepare for the energetic embrace exercise. This time, let both of you move your energy for active penetration. Ouch. What happens as you collide? What sensations arise in you? What feelings? If you were to take it personally, what would you decide about the other person? Laugh.

Now try it with each of you moving to enfold the other passively. What sensations and feelings arise this time? What is the quality of the contact? Do you feel frustrated? What do you decide? How do you respond? Shake it off. Laugh.

Try again with one of you moving to penetrate actively and the other to penetrate passively. What happens? Is any of this painfully familiar?

One more. This time let one of you move actively to enfold as the other enfolds passively. Again notice what confusions, entanglements, frustrations arise and what judgments you would make about this person (and about yourself) if you were "really" moving towards union and embrace under these conditions.

To close the chapter on a more satisfying note, try this **EXERCISE 48:** Stand facing your partner close enough that when you each bend your knees, they come together and touch in a supportive way. Continue the embrace from the knees up. Rest against each other as you hold each other. Experience your emotional and energetic response to this support and intimacy. Separate at will.

Notes

1. I was first introduced to this exercise by Richard Mullens, Ph.D., a trainer for the Bioenergetic Society of Northern California.

2. David Gorman, teaching workshop, Mill Valley, 1984.

3. This exercise is a variation on one I learned from Gerda Alexander, the originator of Eutony, a very subtle approach to body awareness. Her version involves contact through a bamboo stick about nine to 12 inches long. It asks that the energy flow be felt over a distance. Try it.

4. Richard Mullens, Ph.D., taught this exercise at a bioenergetic retreat at Greenwood Lodge, Soquel, California, 1981.

12
But I Can't...
and other Heartfelt Wails

We all experience limits on the amount of pleasure we can feel in being, in touching, in being touched. We also limit our wanting, our reaching, our excitement, our loving. Most of those limits are learned and chosen. Certainly, we aren't usually aware of the choices our culture makes for us or even those of our own choices we made long ago as children about what was possible and appropriate. Our society teaches us that it is "right" or "appropriate" to love or want someone who is beautiful or rich or powerful; then it tells us what *beautiful* is, what *rich* is, what *powerful* is. Such definitions limit our love and our pleasure.

Most people feel better all round when they feel loved and loving. Why wait? Why limit our loving?

EXERCISE 49: What are you waiting for? Bring awareness to the limits of your loving and pleasure. Ask yourself:

Who What and When
. . . do I let myself love?
. . . am I willing to love?
. . . am I willing to want?
. . . am I willing to be excited about?
. . . am I willing to touch?
. . . am I willing to be touched by?
. . . am I willing to reach out for?
. . . am I willing to receive?

EXERCISE 50—The Pillow of Heart's Desire: Sit alone and quiet, or with someone you trust. Put a small cushion in front of you. Visualise the image of your heart's desire resting on the cushion. Be aware of how it will satisfy you. Let yourself reach out and take it. What do you feel? Allow the feelings to expand. Do you let yourself reach? Take? What resistances do you put up to taking the risk of

—knowing what you want?
—knowing that you want it?
—knowing how much you want it?
—taking it?
—taking it in?

In one group which did this exercise, only three people out of seventeen were willing to complete the exercise A few more were willing at least to know what they would reach for, but were unwilling to reach. This is a measure, not of their lack of courage, but of the depth of the risk we feel in wanting from our hearts.

An old Sufi practice suggests that the place to start is by loving yourself. You can begin then to love the stars and the moon, next to love the mountains, the trees and plants and flowers, next the variety of animals, *then* (finally) people, remembering to include yourself among people.

EXERCISE 51: Intend love. Notice when you are loving. Notice where you love. Start there. Love where you can, who or what you can, whenever you can. This "practice" of love strengthens you, as any other practice does. It gives love more room in you.

EXERCISE 52: Make a list of situations in which you let yourself feel "good", e.g., glad, excited, loving, delighted, euphoric, blissful, elated, rapturous. Don't leave *any*thing out. Don't judge anything as silly, inadequate, trivial, or wrong. Notice that in these situations of "feeling good" you are letting your energy expand. Your physical body relaxes; muscle tone increases.

Next notice the kinds of situations in which you feel "bad", e.g., resentful, angry, afraid, disapproving, outraged, anxious, depressed, grieved. Notice that you are contracting your energy (and no doubt your body as well); notice *where* you are contracting, energetically and physically.

EXERCISE 53: In a situation in which you feel good, practise being aware of what is actually happening as you expand. Find your energetic "muscles". Next time you are in a situation in which it is your habit to expand, contract instead, and notice how that affects how you feel. This is a first lesson in feeling what you consciously choose to feel. Now go ahead and let yourself expand as usual. Notice *how* you do it.

EXERCISE 54: A little harder one this time. In a situation in which your habit is to contract, expand instead. (I know this is unexpected. It takes a quantum leap of imagination.) Do

you make difficulties for yourself? Do you say:
> I wouldn't give them the satisfaction . . .
> *Nobody* feels good in this kind of situation . . .
> This is dumb . . .
> This is too hard . . .

Relax; expand anyway. Notice how your feelings change.

EXERCISE 55: Remember a time when you felt exceptionally good. Imagine the situation in all its details: sights and sounds and textures and smells and tastes. Make it real for yourself. Bring it to life. Immerse yourself in the sensations of the experience. Let yourself re-live the good feelings. Notice what happens to your mood and your energy. Notice how mood and energy follow and reflect the reality you are re-creating. Allow the expansion.

Cautiously, do the same exercise using an unpleasant memory. Notice the movement of energy and how your body follows it. Contraction? Compression? Collapse? Allow your awareness to be free of the movement. Watch the contraction (or compression or collapse), and stop it *before* you get stuck. Move your attention back to the pleasant memory. Be very aware of any tendency to decide that the "bad" feeling is more "real" than the "good" feeling. Allow the pleasant feelings reality. Allow the expansion. Contain the energy at a boundary that creates pleasure for you. Pulsate.

You have now done one energetic "push-up". Practise moving from the pleasant memory to the unpleasant one until you can do it easily and smoothly, allowing the rhythm of expansion/contraction/expansion without getting stuck. Pay attention to how the rhythm itself feels. Practise varying the rhythm—long expansion/contraction/expansion like slow deep breaths; quick, lively shifts like the flutter of a giggle. Practise the expansion/contraction/expansion without using the memory. Notice how feeling follows energetic movement.

EXERCISE 56: Review the exercises from "The Energetic Breaths" for diffusion/condensation, collapsing/ballooning, and containment/compression. Find memories that produce these energetic movements. Practise "breathing" back and forth on each axis. Using the memories as a tool until you can expand/contract, condense/diffuse, collapse/balloon, and contain rather than compress—when you choose because you choose.

One common heartfelt wail is, "I don't feel any desire". Probably this is not true. You are probably feeling a lot of desire in (at the moment) rather limited and unsatisfying ways. You may also be assuming that you can't get what you want. You are almost certainly assuming that not getting what you want means you can't be satisfied. That is a particularly deep belief for most people. But I really am saying that you can use the energy of your desire for something you do not have and may never have to experience satisfaction right now.

Start where you are. Avoid judgments. Embrace your ignorance. It is exactly what you don't know that will create a new space for you. So see if you can give up the assumption that you *know* there's something wrong with you; it's not true. You're a human being, and you have limits. You want to expand them. And right there, if you'll notice, you have a desire. Let's use it to move towards satisfaction.

EXERCISE 57: Lying on a comfortable surface, identify the sensation of wanting. Notice what it feels like. If you feel any discomfort, locate the contraction that creates the discomfort. *Where* do you feel the wanting? In your chest? In your belly? In your groin? In your eyes? Wherever it may be, locate the sensation of desire in your body.

That wanting, that desire—however tiny, however much you would like to discount it—is a pocket of charge, a potential pleasure. Practise moving it just a little, as in previous exercises. Notice any assumptions you may have about this particular desire, e.g., that your mother wouldn't approve, that there's no point in wanting something that you can't have, that it doesn't count anyway, that you just *can't* . . . Allow the energy of your desire to expand just a fraction anyway. Notice how you feel. Do you feel the fear of wanting-without-getting? It's an invitation to contract. Okay, contract, but also just a fraction. (Which is easier—expanding or contracting? What's your habit? What's your preference?)

81

Again, allow some expansion into desire. If you feel the need to contract, do, just a little; then expand again. Your physical body will follow this energetic movement, relaxing and contracting also. Like the chicken and the egg, your mind, your physical body, and your energetic body are all leading each other. Expand a little, contract a little. It's like breathing, in and out. Allow the rhythm of pulsation. Begin to relax into the rhythm itself. Pleasure may begin to arise as you simply allow the experience of pulsation. Allow it as much as you can. Allow some of the sound of your desire to express itself.

Now begin to move the energy of your wanting around a bit in your body. If you feel the longing in your heart, move it out into your arms and hands. (Remember intention, visualisation, breath, movement.) Notice, as you do this, that a desire to reach out begins to arise. Let yourself reach out. Reach towards what you want even though you can't see it or feel it there. (Be attentive and merciful towards any feelings of fear, humiliation, contempt; you may have been taught that it's shameful or stupid to want what you "can't" have.)

Now move the energy downwards into your belly, pelvis, legs, feet. Use any of the exercises and hints in the chapter "Getting It There" to help you. Be aware of your intention, visualise the movement, let physical movement arise to assist direction, and breathe in the direction you want things to go. Ground your feet and breathe pelvically. Feel your wanting in belly and legs; feel it in the *ground* if you can.

Don't panic. I know it's a lot to coordinate, but you learned to drive a stick shift, and this is no more complicated. Give yourself a pat and three gold stars for having come this far. Relax. Let what's happening happen.

Now move some of that energy up into your face and eyes. Feel the sensations of desire in your mouth and tongue and lips and eyes. Now relax all effort. Let down. Let yourself rest on the inner column of energy you have created. Sound your surrender. As you release yourself from effort, you will experience a movement towards orgasm.

It may seem small. Avoid judgment. Judging the movement to be small is a decision to contract, and then you have it all to do again. Actually this movement of life in response to itself is a kind of miracle. We all have a phenomenal compulsion to improve the miracle.

Any desire at all can be used in just this fashion to stretch your capacity to experience pleasure. The desire for a lover is often strongest for most people; but, if you will give up judging things to be trivial, you can use the desire for a warm bath, for a sack of chocolate truffles, or for the chairmanship of General Motors to release yourself into pleasure. It's the energy, not the object, that allows orgasm. You can use the desire for pleasure itself to lead you to satisfaction.

Sometimes loving people is very difficult. Perhaps you say, "I can love the plants and animals, but . . ." Okay. Once again, begin by eliminating old judgments. Get rid of the "but". Making a negative judgment is a decision to contract. (Incidentally, making a positive judgment is *not* usually a decision to expand, but to balloon.) All judgments diminish life and diminish pleasure in being. So. With plants and animals, you let yourself feel loving. Fine, let's do it.

EXERCISE 58: Choose a flower or a tree or your favourite cat. Trees are good to try this with first. They're stable, they hold still, and they have loads of energy. As you would with a human partner, pick a distance from the tree that allows you to feel the energetic presence of the tree and still to experience yourself as separate. Eyes open or closed, practise forming the energy column along your spine. Then allow yourself to feel your love for the tree. Let your energy flow forward to merge with the energy of the tree. Continue to feel loving as you withdraw your energy from the tree and feel your separateness. Be separate with an open heart. (Notice that with your heart open, you can contain your energy quite close to your physical body without getting stuck in contraction.) Again merge and separate. Do this as many times as you like; the pulsation will build charge. Make sounds that express and expand your experience. Feeling the pleasure of this pulsation, you may want to enhance it by breathing pelvically. As you feel your love for the tree and feel charge building within you and between you, you may find in yourself a desire for union. Allow flow between your heart and groin and *from* both heart and groin towards the tree. Then, as you next flow towards the tree, open yourself also to receive the energy of the tree. Surrender. Allow yourself to feel the touching, as you either enfold or penetrate the tree. You will experience a movement towards orgasm.

You can vary this exercise in any of the ways noted in the chapter, "The Energetic Embrace". Consider a knee hug with the tree. Do the exercise again with any creature you love or with whom you are willing to experience union. Notice how very different they are and that they, too, may have energetic preferences. Consider including people in the great range of creatures.

13

Control and Abandon

Have you ever thought to wonder to yourself what orgasm actually is? I'll bet you never said to yourself, "Why, it's a spontaneous, reflexive re-distribution of energy". At least I hope not.[1] But orgasm *is* a spontaneous, reflexive re-distribution of energy; and, *because* it is, orgasm is not limited to genital release, nor to sexual contact as a stimulus. It means that sneezes can be orgasmic. It means that the tension you collect between your shoulder blades can release orgasmically. It means that, whenever you have extra energy collected somewhere and you're willing simply to surrender to the tendency of that energy to *move*, you can allow yourself orgasm.

I mentioned to you before Don Juan's description of the aware person "walking the line between control and abandon". It is the balance between controlling our responses and abandoning ourselves to them that allows "spontaneous, reflexive re-distribution of energy". The moment we surrender to the mutual demands of control and abandon, we move towards an orgasmic reponse to being. These experiences arise not from abandoning the body for La-la-land but instead from going deeper and deeper into bodily experience.[2]

Containment itself is a model of this "walking the line". We control in maintaining the boundary we have chosen, but we also abandon ourselves to the impulse to expand: over and over, we expand and return to the boundary. Over and over, we balance control and abandon. This balance *is* the pulsation. And in that moment when we surrender to the balanced forces—without choosing one over the other—orgasm becomes inevitable.

All of the exercises in the book are invitations to find and walk this line, but any exercise anywhere, any activity anywhere can be engaged in this way.

Notes

1. This may be my favourite bit of jargon in the world, along with *bracts of the involucre, torquing the dura,* and *archaic superego introjects.*

2. Thanks for the reminder to mention this goes to Walt Watman, Ph.D., bioenergetic analyst.

14
The Lover Within

All we have learned so far leads to this, to begin to experience the possibility of your own life, moving in you, as orgasmic.

How, then, to invite the lover within? If you experience yourself as the vessel that life penetrates, which is so, then all you have to do is to let that penetration touch you as fully and deeply as possible in every moment. Of course, this "all" is more than a minor step. The psycho-orgastic exercise introduced later in this chapter is in itself one invitation, which can be extended again and again.

For me, the way in has been to approach any place where I am withholding energy—keeping it in stasis—whether in my unexpressed longing for union, or my fear that I won't have enough money, or my anger at the man who didn't love me as I wanted him to. Wherever there is energy in stasis, there is an engorgement, a honeypot waiting to flow. I do whatever I know how to allow the energy into my awareness, to encourage it to move, and then to surrender to it. Gradually it becomes orgasmic.

To the extent that we limit our possibilities for pleasure and orgasm to genital sexuality, we don't even consider these other possibilities—or they sound abstract and far-off. For me, nothing is so exciting as to imagine that *life* is my lover—and is *always* courting me. To relate to life in that way is a challenge and a surrender that invites me deeper into being alive in every moment that I can manage it.

Step by step by step, I have said, "Hey, something is interfering with my enjoying being here. What the hell is it? And what can I do about it?" Each time I confront one of these inner insistent negativities—"Oh, I can't have that!" "Life's just not like that." "I'll never forgive him!" "That's not possible!"—I open the energy package of such an assumption; I open myself to new gifts of energy and pleasure and excitement. Whenever I find one of the places in which I hold energy bound up in an assumption of what is and what can be, then I know there's another gift to be unwrapped. It may take me some time to locate what it is and where I'm holding on. But it's always an insistence, a contraction, that stands between me and a fuller pleasure in being: not that I can't have X, but that I insist I *must* have it before I allow myelf to feel pleasure in being; not that I don't have X, but that I *assume* that I can't have it and *hold* energy in the assumption. When I can trust opening past the possibility of having X to the possibility of satisfaction with *or* without it, then my capacity for pleasure expands.

My deepest experience of this process (so far) came along a few years ago. I went through a patch of misery that July and came into August just surging inwardly. First, all I could feel was pressure and discomfort. Then I decided that the pressure was my longing for union. I said, "Oh, no, I've worked on this *before*, why do I have to do this again"—complain, bitch, moan, whine, and on and on. Finally, I directed my attention inward beyond what I knew; and I said, "I would like a resolution of this; I don't know how it *spozed* to happen. I'm totally ignorant. Assume I'm retarded, only let's just *do* something about this contraction, ok?" The next day I woke up having decided to stop labelling the event. I decided to accept that there was a lot of energy moving in me—or wanting to move; I decided to give up calling it "longing" and attaching the energy to a certain desired outcome. I decided that from then on, as much as I could, I would relate to the energy simply as energy, as life; I would give it as much space as I could, and let it move as much as I could. Then there came a period of about a week or ten days when I felt as if I were being pressed and stretched open, again and again—like giving birth inwards. The experience tested my trust of myself and my friends. I had to ask, "Whom do I trust myself to? How far do I trust myself to reveal that this is going on with me?" I looked around for those people and spent a lot of time with them. I told them I wasn't going to censor much and might make some unexpected sounds. One of these great floods of energy would come through, and I would gasp. Since I had given up censoring, I could hear that it sounded like a pleasure sound. But I was still separating myself from the experience. I began to trust myself to reduce the distance; I began to surrender. As I did, the sensations I felt went from neutral to warm to ecstatic—still the experience of being stretched and filled with a great flowing, rising wave. I didn't, and don't, know what to call it but orgasmic.

I had that experience with longing, and my longing was satisfied from within. I was no longer longing painfully for a mate. Then a maniacal anger at an old lover came up—a desire (this time a desire to rend him limb from limb)—and I thought, "Well, if I can expand to cleanse my longing, why not this rage?" So I did, and the anger cooled. The energy was there but without the same obsessive (that is, compressive) feeling to it. Again, in the process there was a welling, surging pleasurable release of energy throughout my body. Then I did it with fear about money, releasing more pleasure. (I'm still working on that one—one of the more persuasive myths.)

What I've learned so far is that whenever I find a holding in myself, an insistence on a certain condition or outcome, and I can separate the *energy* of my insistence from that outcome, pleasure arises. Often, in the beginning, it's more pleasure than I know what to do with—than I can "contain" literally—and so I may experience it as discomfort. I have to go easy, remember to be patient and merciful with myself, and remind myself to respect my limits and to trust. Gradually I stretch; gradually I am big enough.

EXERCISE 59: This exercise involves about nine minutes of charging through movement and breath, followed by an opportunity to release the gathered energy back through the whole system. People have described this experience as "orgasmic", as "being filled with light", as "a funny thing like being in control and out of control at the same time", as a disappointment because "nothing happened", as confusing, as annoying, as a revelation, as a "grateful wholeness". Give yourself permission not to anticipate, not to expect, not to judge. Allow what happens, respecting your limits and stretching them. Above all, try not to improve the miracle.

You'll need to have a watch with a sweep hand or a stopwatch or some other tool that counts seconds. Best to have an assistant to watch the time for you, at least to begin with. The charging sequence of the exercise is made up of nine variations on pelvic breathing,[1] as follows: Sit on the floor, resting back on your hands. Place your feet, soles together, out in front of you, knees open. Breathe pelvically in this position for one minute. Let the breath find its own rhythm as your attention moves into your pelvis. When the first minute is up, simply bring your feet half way to your groin and continue the pelvic breathing. Sounds, of course. Be aware of the sensations that begin to arise as you collect energy in your pelvis. After the second minute bring your feet up further, as close as you comfortably can, towards your pelvis. Breathe pelvically for another minute. Make sounds; relax into the experience of collecting and containing this energy. After this third minute, move your feet back out to the first position and lower yourself onto your elbows. Breathe pelvically for another three minutes, moving your feet through the three positions of closeness. This brings you up to six minutes. (Don't let your head fall back in this position, though it may be a temptation; heads are heavy, and you could strain your neck.) Lower yourself down onto your back and breathe for another three minutes, again moving your legs through the three positions. At this point, you have a number of choices.

To begin with, try simply lifting your knees slowly as you did in Exercise 44. This time, you'll probably notice a major difference due to the increased charge you've created by the nine minutes of pelvic breathing. You may experience very intense vibration beginning in your thighs and expanding outwards throughout your body. When you find the place of most openness (and if your limits permit), rest in that place and allow yourself to surrender to the experience. You can vary the placement of your feet (from close together to far apart) to vary the flavour and texture of the experience. You can also press down lightly on your feet to shift the direction of flow or to assist yourself to move through some interruption of the flow, either down through your legs or up through your body. As the vibration touches on certain places in your body—your diaphragm, for example, or your chest or throat or eyes—you're likely to find that strong feelings arise and ask for expression. Try to allow them to be part of the pulsation. Make sounds to express the feelings.

It's very important for you to remember that no one will have the same experience of this exercise. You may want to open your arms and reach out as the vibration reaches your chest (or to encourage the vibration to reach further into you). You may want to laugh or sob. You may want to growl with frustration.

When you've gone as deeply into the exercise as you want to at this time—or when you simply need to rest yourself—turn to your left side and rest there, allowing your energy to move and your awareness to be at one with the movement.

One or two of the more important possible variations include doing the exercise to music and/or including an additional charging and opening exercise at the end of the pelvic breathing. Music is delightful with this exercise, and you can to some extent "program" the direction of the experience by the choice of music. Try it with Olatunji's *Drums of Passion, Variations on a Theme of Thomas Tallis* by Vaughn Williams, Pachelbel's *Canon*, Mozart's *Requiem*, practically anything by the Moody Blues, or some lovely spacey thing by Steve Halpern or Schawkie Roth or Constance Denby. Anything. One caution: be sure you like the music and the way you respond to it.

One of the things you are almost certain to feel as you reach the edge of your current limits with this exercise is pressure. This pressure you feel is life, the energy of your being. Often we are brought up to repress this life and, not to identify with it, but to identify with our resistance to it.

In going into yourself through this exercise, you can choose where you place your conciousness—your "self". You can be the pressure or the container of the pressure. If you like—and it's a very pleasant thing to do—you can "be" the container. You can identify with your body as a vessel, opening and stretching to receive life, the lover within. You can allow yourself to be filled with that life, the pressure of it expanding and filling you. If you relax down onto that pressure, life will support you—as water, moving through a hose under pressure, lifts it. If you surrender to this moment, you will move towards orgasm. If you clamp down, contract and say, "I'm doing it wrong," and "I can't let it through," and all the other thngs we say, you will be uncomfortable. If you expand, even a fraction, you will feel life there, pressing into you, through you—as much as you can *now*. You can say, "Ah, good, let go." Surrender. Relax down altogether onto that supporting pressure. There will be a movement towards orgasm, no matter what the stimulus. At first the movement may be incomplete. Certainly, in the beginning, I myself felt almost no movement at all. I was very creative with harsh things to say to myself about myself. The more I learned to decline these judgments, the more movement arose. And so, a little deeper, a little more free, a little more filled and surrendered. Now, during all the moments I can let myelf remember to let go, I have a love relationship with life instead of a struggle.

One of the things taught in tantra is that we are each of us *both* poles of energy—the active and the passive, the penetrative and enfolding. Within each of us is the other pole of our conscious identification. Just as when we unite energetically with another person, we can be penetrative or enfolding, active or passive with our energies, so within ourselves we can move to union from either pole. We can identify with the vessel—the "cup"—of the body and lift it to be filled by life. Or we can move identity to the energy itself, "be" that which presses the vessel to fullness. We can imagine the body as our beloved, and be as gentle, as assertive, and as pleasantly insistent as a courting lover.

Throughout this book I have emphasised that a person can build charge deliberately—in the pelvis or in some other part of the body—and then release it. This experience is—can become—orgasmic. That's why I refer to it as *the lover within*. It becomes possible to extend to many of our internal responses the surrender that permits orgasm.

Because we experience ourselves energetically as living in a container, the physical body, we feel ourselves as enclosed. Usually our experience of our own energy is fairly static, not very flowing except when we're making love (and not always then). It is possible to learn how to allow your energy to flow in response to many situations and events, internal and external.

Desire itself can trigger orgasm as long as the wanting is allowed to expand without regard to *getting*. By dissolving your attachment to the outcome, the energy you have invested in the object becomes available to flow. You can become that flow orgasmically.

Though we experience ourselves as enclosed, the energy of the universe (of "all that is") is without boundaries. Apparent boundaries are not real boundaries energetically. If you can find a way to channel, to release, through your body, those energies that come from life "beyond you", then you have the sensation of the lover within.

According to Indian and Tibetan schools of tantra, people usually identify with one aspect—one pole—of their own energy (see "The Energetic Embrace") and hold the opposite polarity separate (and usually unconscious). For example, as I am female and identify with being female, I am likely to experience my inner energy as male. I can allow myself to unite with that inner energy. It is clear that this is another question of boundaries—where we make them, place them, experience them. In this case, we can engage our own inner boundaries in merging and separating, as we have before with a partner. Tantricas—students of tantra—learn to open themselves to the opposite pole of energy in their partners and in themselves and to become one with that opposite. This has nothing to do with gender; it has to do with the aspect of your energy that you identify with.

In certain Tibetan spiritual practices, the student is encouraged to visualise in great detail the divine lover and move into union with that beloved. This practice helps the student to move beyond her current boundaries and expectations of what she is. With full involvement, this union also becomes orgasmic.

Probably the most famous of modern schools to deal with this inner polarity is the psychology of C. G. Jung. Jung talks about this encounter with the opposite within us in terms of *anima* and *animus*. As he describes these "complexes" we each hold unconscious within us, it is clear that we encounter them in our lovers. We first encounter our inner lover in the mirror of the world; we project our own inner opposite onto the men and women we meet. Jung speaks of the feminine energy of the man as his *anima*. A man's tendency to project his "soul energy" outside of himself blurs his perception of women as individuals. This leads to frustrated talk about how "all women are alike". Women, Jung says, have within them a masculine energy called the *animus*. They also project this part of themselves, making mirrors of the men around them. The more they insist on trying to find outside themselves the "ghost lover" within, the more these "reflections" confuse and limit what they can know of the men they love.

Jung sees the encounter with this opposite within us and its integration into the personality as an important stage of growth, one that cannot be avoided without damage to the individual. But, as he describes it, this stage is "personal" and preliminary to the greater union described in tantra. In a recently published article in the Jungian journal *Chiron*,[2] Nathan Schwartz-Salant bravely and carefully describes the movement towards energetic union that sometimes occurs in the therapeutic relationship. He describes it in strictly Jungian terms and doesn't have the concept of the energy body to draw on. Yet it is clear that he recognises there is a somatic and energetic element in this impulse to union. This he refers to as the "subtle body". He also points out that a lot of "sexual acting out" that happens in the therapeutic situation—not to mention the greater cauldron of life—is a fumbling attempt to allow meaningful energetic union.

In these exercises, we engage the energy body directly in a movement towards a similar integration. Beyond self-union, or through self-union, lies the possibility of a greater union. Tilopa, the Tibetan, speaks of it in his *Song of Mahamudra*:

Millions and millions of times deeper,
millions and millions of times higher, is Mahamudra.
It is a total orgasm with the Whole, with the universe.
It is melting into the source of Being.[3]

He is talking about an orgasmic union with the whole of what is. Mahamudra—the great gesture—is orgasm as a response simply to being. What he implies is that the universe as a whole is in a constant experience of orgasm—the gathering and release of charge. In always asserting our separateness and not knowing how to receive the whole, we create barriers that prevent a continuing movement towards and through orgasm. It is, after all, beyond conception to contain all that is. The Indian poet Kabir referred to it as "the ocean falling into the drop".

Sometimes people ask in puzzlement how or why enlightened masters "renounce" sex. They don't. It isn't a matter of giving it up; sex loses its relevance. The charge between you and everything-that-is is so much greater than it can be between you and another little bit of what is that sex is a damp squib in comparison.[4]

In tantra as a sexual meditation, each lover regards the other not only as an individual but as a focus, a channel, for embracing all that is. That's why tantricas say that sexuality is the gateway, the way in, towards mahamudra. Nonpersonal sexual charge moves naturally into love, into grace, and into gladness; that movement is inevitable as long as you keep opening more and more.

We are separate and not separate. We are the balance between control and abandon. There is a constantly shifting but inexhaustible source of energy that is just "is-ness". Getting access to that is an adventure in choosing boundaries and surrendering to pulsation.

It means letting go of your insistence on who you are and what you are and how life is. It also involves questions of how much you can stand. How much of the whole energy-of-what-is can this infinitesimal nexus bear to contain? People can go mad. We make boundaries so that we can feel separate and move coherently through the world; it's part of our necessary natural growth to do that. In doing it, we forget the secret, which is that we are not separate.

What is, is inseparable. When you can open the inner door and let that energy flow, you can nourish yourself directly.

Respect your limits. Love your limits; they protect you from an abundance so immense it can be intolerable. If, however, you stretch your limits also, you will move in the direction of receiving and becoming unconditional love.

Notes

1. I first learned this charging sequence from Michael Conant, Ph.D., then head trainer of the Bioenergetic Society of Northern California; he had it from someone in Oregon.

2. Nathan Schwartz-Salant, "Archetypal Factors Underlying Sexual Acting Out in the Transference/Countertransference Process", from *Chiron*, 1984, pp. 1–30.

3. Tilopa, *Song of Mahamudra*, as quoted in *Only One Sky* by B. S. Rajneesh, p. 5.

15
Movement, Breath, and Sound

The approach to emotional and energetic freedom of choice presented in this section got its start in 1984 when a doctor friend, Bonnie Scott Steuble, sent me an article from the *San Francisco Chronicle* about work that Paul Ekman and Bob Levinson were doing on the physiology of emotion. In particular, the article described experiments they were doing with young actors, asking them to move various muscles in their faces in particular ways and notice how they felt. This was right up my alley as I had not only been trained as an actress, but in the course of my studies of somatics and somatic psychotherapy, I had come to have a practical grasp of how we create our feeling states. So, on impulse, I gave them a call. Bob and I had pizza and talked, and I shamelessly said that I knew quite a lot about what they were studying. I don't think he quite believed me, but he was kind enough to ask me if I would like to observe when Joe de Rivera, a noted phenomenological psychologist from Clarke University, went through their procedures. Yes, indeed I would. Actually, when the day came, the thought of the long trip into San Francisco was daunting, but then they asked me if I would, after all, go through the protocol myself, and I was hooked.

I never did see Joe's run; there was some need to preserve my purity for my run through of the experiment. When it came time for my turn, I did about as well as anyone else on the main part of the procedure; that is, I could move the indicated muscles well enough and identify the corresponding feelings. But I was no better at it than anyone else. What came next began a very interesting and, for me, profitable association. As part of the protocol, each person was asked if they could feel what they wanted to feel simply by choosing to feel it. I think this was in the protocol because of the notion that actors can, through sensory recall—sense memory—feel what they choose. Actually, it is far from being the case. What is recalled is a kind of ghost that can serve as a trigger if the actor is very skillful.

When Paul asked me if I could feel what I chose to feel, I said yes. I know he didn't believe me. So we started out with anger. Can you feel anger? He asked. Yes. Okay, do it. So I did. He came dashing in to put out the fire. Wait, wait, he said, we have to recalibrate the instruments, you're off the scale! What a satisfaction to have surprised him.

After that, we did sadness, fear, disgust, and happiness. My so cooperative body was a bit in shock. My body wanted to know why on earth we had done this. I knew I would have to come up with a good story. In fact, when Paul and Bob asked if I would be willing to explore this further with them, I said a lot would depend on whether I could do it without damaging the cooperative relationship of body and conscious intention. It had taken me years to cultivate that close, immediate alliance between my conscious intention and my bodily willingness to respond, and I didn't want to damage it by asking of my body responses it thought stupid.

In any case, somewhere along the line Paul asked me if I could teach other people how to be able to feel what they chose to feel. I said, let me think about it. I did, and after a few days came back to him with six key words: *movement, breath, sound, intention, consent,* and *surrender*. He organized a weekend workshop for some friends and we tried it out in practice. It worked.

Since then, the observation that feeling states arise simultaneously with and as the direct expression of how we are *moving* (or not moving), how we are *breathing* (or not breathing), how we are allowing expressive *sound* (or suppressing it) has proved central to the way that I work as a somaticist and psychotherapist and also to the practice of meditation as I now understand it.

In order to take practical advantage of knowing that movement, breath, and sound are the creators of our feeling states, the other three words come into play: *intention, consent, surrender*. We have to intend to feel something; we have to consent to move, breathe, and make sound in the ways associated with that state; we have to surrender to the effects we are creating.

This, like everything else I am sharing with you, has a practical intention: to give you the tools you need to begin to have more choice over what you are feeling and to feel good more of the time.

Before We Begin: Anger, Fear, and Sadness

For most people, anger or fear or sadness—or more than one of them—is a state they spend more time in than they would like. They get *stuck* in them like boots in mud or superglue on fingers. The feelings seem to come by themselves, often for no reason that we can notice, and sometimes they hang around for days, making us miserable.

When I was studying Redecision Therapy with George Thomson from 1975 to 1978,[1] one of the most dazzling pieces of information he brought to us was what anger, fear, and sadness were *for*—whyever would we feel them at all? In case this information has passed you by, I'd like to share it with you. For one reason, because it is the beginning of meeting these old enemies as friends, and, for another, because, of all the things I learned from George (and there were many), few have been so clearly helpful to me in working out what the hell was going on when I felt overwhelmed by feeling.

Anger

First, let's have a working definition: *Anger* is the energized frustration we feel when we want to change something and, so far, we can't. This same energy arises *whenever* we want to change something—doesn't matter what. It is the energy we set in motion to do *anything*—cross the room, turn on the light switch, close the window, climb a mountain, turn on the tv, sing a song. We only *call* it anger when we encounter a difficulty in doing what we want to do.

So one thing I'd like you to carve into your bedpost and look at every day, morning and night, especially if you have troubles with anger—feeling too much or too little—is that anger is not at all the same thing as wanting to hurt someone. It is only, but essentially, the energy we access to create change. Only under extreme conditions of threat and powerlessness does our natural need to change things become distorted into a wish to do harm.

So why, if anger is helpful and even essential, is it such a pain—in the neck, in the gut, in the ass, wherever we store the energy we are *not* using to change things? Mostly, anger becomes painful when we are wanting to change the past or the future rather than the present. We get stuck in time. We still feel unsafe because some relative was unreliable or violent, and we are still trying to make him or her be different—

even when they aren't there any more. Your body doesn't know that things have changed, so it has a hair trigger in regards to certain people or situations. Because we get stuck in trying—and trying and trying—to resolve a past that is already over and done with, we go on feeling feelings that were appropriate in the past but are out of place—out of time—now.

To be revved up to change things that no longer need to be changed or to change things that can't, at the moment, be changed, is nothing but exhausting. It depletes our resources of energy and often makes it nearly impossible to notice what we *can* change.

FEAR

Working definition: *Fear* is the energized set of sensations that tells us something dangerous is present and that we need either to confront it vigorously or to move away from it—now and briskly, thank you. Whether we confront it or move away, the fear signals dissolve and the energy remains. If we move away, we feel we could run for days or leap effortlessly to a high branch. Which, of course, is what the energy is for, historically. Out there on the edge between forest and veldt, there were a lot of creatures bigger and stronger than us who thought we'd make a good meal. We needed to be able to put on short bursts of speed or jump uncommonly high to save ourselves. Even now when we move without inhibition to confront or flee what threatens us, the sensations change from fear to exhilaration. The energy is the same. The sensations of chronic fear persist only when we feel there is something dangerous present that we dare not confront or leave behind.

The fear signals, like the anger signals, are essential. We have to have the information they provide, or we won't notice that we are in danger. Or, rather, we might notice—ah, I see, a deadly poisonous bank manager—but without juice, without the motivation to move away from the danger. (Or crack it a good one over the knuckles, if that's appropriate.)

It does no good to feel in danger *all* the time. Your perception is then inaccurate—it simply isn't true, not even in war—and your capacity to perceive and respond to what is actually happening is reduced. The inaccuracy of perception puts you in greater danger—if there is any—than if you were relaxed and alert.

But fear signals, also, get stuck in time. Our body goes on telling us the dangerous mother/father is there long after they have changed or died, long after we are no longer the vulnerable child who *couldn't* leave. So, oftentimes, we live our lives assuming we have no more choice to leave a threatening or unpleasant situation than a three-year-old child. That is a neurochemical assumption that asserts itself whenever the past appears to be happening now. Whenever we imagine a future bound by the past. Whenever the present is muddied over by past experiences *as if they were true now.*

SADNESS

Working definition: *Sadness*, especially accompanied by weeping, is the means by which we adjust to loss. It permits a re-regulation of the body's homeostasis (its stable steady-state level of functioning) to accommodate new conditions—gain as well as loss, actually.

As with fear and anger, sadness provides an essential function. It is one of our most effective ways of letting the past be passed, so the present can be cleanly and clearly whatever it is, and we can respond to it *as it is*, rather than assuming it is just the past all over again. But we have to let the past be past, let the weeping be whole-hearted and sweep through the body like a tide. We have to notice that the past *is* past. When we refuse our grief, or refuse to let it complete itself, then our knowledge of the past passing remains conceptual: yes, my true love has died, and that was 15 years ago, but I'll start eating soon. The body itself must recognize the loss is over, no longer happening.

The body experiences only the present moment, but if its perceptions are stuck in time, it will experience some *other* moment as present, often over and over. The strong, whole-body pulsations of weeping help to wash away the past and let its story become part of the present without harm.

All of the exercises that follow support greater choice over the qualities of movement and breath and sound that we bring to our daily living. The more choice we *know* we have in how we breathe, how we move, and what sounds we make, the less we are stuck in time. We are then more free to feel anger when our need to change something *in the present* is frustrated, fear when we need to confront or flee some danger *now*, sadness when loss arises in our *present* life. We are also free to spend more and more time in states of well-being.

Getting on with Movement, Breath, and Sound

ANGER PLAY

I don't really mean this to be a cookbook: breathe thus and so, stomp your feet and holler, let yourself go into this combination of movement, breath, and sound, and you will *be* angry. In fact it's true—and we will be learning some of these circus tricks—but that's not the most helpful aspect of what we will be doing. I would like to lead you through some experiments that will let you learn directly—so that, by and by, you really *know* through and through—that you are always choosing how you feel through the ways you breathe, move, and make sound. This is true even though you are very unlikely to be *conscious* of choosing—at this point, your body is choosing for you. Most of us live in this way from one feeling habit to another, one reaction to another, but once you really know that you make what you feel and that there is something you can do about what you are making, you will be half-way home. Half-way to moving with some freedom out of feelings that belong to the past. Half-way to developing a new habit of well-being.

Ok. So let's try a few of the circus tricks. If we can kickstart some of the common garden variety "bad" feelings whenever we want to, we can start standing free of them. We will carry on from those experiments to initiating a few states that are more pleasant.

Please do not choose to start with a feeling that you are commonly stuck in!

We will start with how to feel angry "just because"—which is the same thing as beginning to notice you don't *have* to do this, and the same thing as beginning to notice that you *can* do this now even if it was dangerous when you were little.

EXERCISE 60: Let your lower jaw come forward so your lower teeth are in front of your upper teeth (notice this is a *movement*). Begin to breathe so that your whole chest rises and falls with each breath you take (a style of *breathing*). As you breathe in this way with your lower jaw forward, growl or howl (this is the *sound* part). Do this without thinking about it much, just for the hell of it, and without holding back or "watching" yourself, for about 20 or 30 seconds. It probably won't take that long for you to notice that you are angry. For some, the effect will be instantaneous because there is no strong inhibition against being angry—or against feeling slightly silly. If fear is your main sticky feeling, you may need to find a safe place or a good friend in order to feel safe enough to let yourself do this the first time or two.

Notice that when you stop breathing, moving, and making sounds in this particular way, you very quickly come out of feeling angry. In fact, as your nervous system gets more flexible and more "current," the feeling of anger will stop instantly.

EXERCISE 61: Breathe, move, and make sound as you did in the exercise above. In addition, let your arms rise and fall with the breath (*movement*) and make fists (*ditto*). Jump up and down (*ditto*).

This is the full flame-out primate version. You may feel a fuller surge of anger, followed by feelings of pleasure and grateful silliness. If you feel like laughing, please do. The full version really requires a tree branch for complete satisfaction.

EXERCISE 62: Begin to do the first anger exercise, but pretend you have to do it so that nobody notices. Let the movement, breath, and sound—and all the energy and impetus of them—be present but very, very small.

This way of being angry may be *much* more familiar than the open versions, especially the full-blooded primate announcement, "I object!" (with tree branch, of course). When we feel we have to disguise our objections in this way, especially when we suppress our need to take action to change things, we create stagnant pockets of energy and fluid that predispose us to feel bad and can, in the long run, lead to such conditions as arthritis and ulcers.

FEAR PLAY

Now, any time you fancy the experiment, you can make the movements, the breaths, and the sounds that create fear. If fear is a common state for you, put this off until you are less convinced that life is always dangerous. It's also a good idea to have a place where you can run off some of the energy you have generated.

As we said about anger, learning that you can kickstart the energies of "fight or flight" just because you want to is the same as beginning to know that you can let yourself have those energies and responses when you truly need them *and* that you don't have to be convinced by an old habit.

EXERCISE 63: Open your eyes wide and let your eyebrows go up. Begin to breathe in short fast gasps high in your chest. Let your body twist slightly as if you are about to run. Say, "No no no!"

As with the basic exercise to make anger, try this without withholding, thinking, or watching for twenty or thirty seconds and see where you get to. If you are practiced in feeling fear, the arising of fear sensations may be instantaneous. If feeling fear is something you don't allow yourself often, you may have to play at it longer.

If feeling scared is scary for you, come out of it immediately. Take your breath deeper in your body, stamp your feet, stand upright, make fists, and glare around threateningly. If you can bring yourself to do it, bare your teeth. Your body needs to do these things to make sure any other primates in the neighborhood (visible or not) know that you are no pushover. When you have established your willingness to protect yourself, come further down into calm if you want or need to, using any of the exercises in the section called "Tolerance for Calm."

EXERCISE 64: If the surge of energy associated with being frightened doesn't in itself unnerve you, try the further experiment of using the energy you feel to run for half a mile or so—you may feel like you are soaring.

EXERCISE 65: The other half of "flight" is "fight." You may find it very strengthening to use the fear juices you have made to punch a punching bag or bite on a rump steak. If you do this without worry or watching, it is likely that strong pleasure sensations will come with the information that you are strong and willing to protect yourself.

Just to state the obvious, the purpose of these exercises is not to scare yourself (except literally) but to show you the sorts of movement, breath, and sound that go with feeling afraid so that *you can do something else if you want to.* This is especially true in regards to the habit of fear with which so many of us live. However, it is also true that, when danger is real and immediate, we need to feel willing and able to run like billy ned or, when necessary, strike out to protect ourselves.

SADNESS PLAY

Now we come to the last of our freedom experiments with "bad" feelings—how to feel sad "just because." As with anger and fear, our intention is not to dig deeper grooves for old feeling habits but to feel from the inside out how they get established and how we can begin to step free of them.

EXERCISE 66: Sit so that your chest is a little collapsed. Let each outbreath be a bit longer than its inbreath. Breathe more with your belly than your chest. Gently tense and lift the inner corners of your eyebrows. Let your eyes glaze over and go inward. Sigh with each breath.

Within 20-30 seconds, or less if you have the habit of sadness, your eyes will moisten and the fluid in your mouth will increase. If there is some loss you haven't resolved yet, consider letting yourself move into free weeping. (If you do, it will involve a much more open breath, sobbing sounds, and a whole-body surrender to the pulsations of grief.) If you have no current need for sadness, bring your spine flexibly upright, breathe freely, and smile.

For many of us, habits of fear, anger, and sadness are central to how we structure the time and meaning of our lives and the quality of how we spend our days. In the next section, we begin to look at what we can do instead.

As my friend Susan once said, with breathtaking clarity, "But if I give up being unhappy, what will I do with my *time*!?!"

Let's see.

Tolerance for Calm

One of the odd things people have occasionally asked me is, "Does all this mean we won't be able to feel our feelings?" Well, no, of course not. Emphatically not, even. What it does mean is that *if you care to*, you can change what you are feeling pretty much when you want to. Certainly it doesn't mean that you will always want to. Sometimes, as we've seen, anger, fear, and sadness serve us well in essential ways, and the energies and changes they generate are to our benefit. Other times, ok, we're angry or something for no very good reason, but it's easier to ride it out than to actively change what we are feeling. (Still, I would bet a bundle that to feel something from this perspective will already have changed movement, breath, and sound and, therefore, what you are feeling.)

What is often behind the strange question, "Does all this mean we won't be able to feel our feelings?" is something much deeper. In the West, we take our turbulence to be a sign of aliveness. Many of us fear that not to be in a state of turbulence means to be or feel deadened. Those of us who grew up often under threat, for example, may confuse the sensations of dread with the experience of *being* itself. If some such thing is true for you—whether you have wedded your being to anger, fear, or sadness—it may take some time to test the ground of well-being and discover that you haven't lost your self when you "rest down"[2] out of agitation into calmness and well-being as your more ordinary state.

Richardson's Vigilance

My friend Tony Richardson is a doctor and a shrink as well as one of the finest somaticists, somatic psychotherapists, and Tibetan Buddhist practitioners I know. It's a gaudy but reliable combination and leads to our having some very uncommon conversations. One of these took place some time back when we were discussing the physiological, somatic, and experiential differences between depression and despair. Now, obviously, this is a complex and thorny issue, but something very valuable came out of our talk. At the end of our conversation, we decided, as a working hypothesis, that despair was the long-term effect of feeling that one could *never* really safely let down, rest down, because there was no felt ground of holding and safety—no love presence. No true mother's lap or father's strong arms in all the world.

106

When this sort of experience gets structured into our nervous system as we grow up, we can come to feel that letting down itself—even the impulse to let down—is what triggers danger to arise. What we end up with is a nervous system that *won't* rest down because the resting state is felt to be dangerous.

When we are in the early years of our adulthood, we may not feel this very much except as a drive to create safety—by creating love or isolation or power or money or whatever else we may have associated with everything finally being ok. Later, when we begin to feel the fatigue of being driven in this way and really *want* to let down, we find that we can't. Not for itself, not *as things are*. So we rely on secondary conditions to compensate—we may eat more or drink more or have sex more or buy more or take control more, trying to create a situation in which we will have at least the illusion of resting down. The more effort we put into trying to make things "ok" enough to rest down, the more fatigued we get, and the more a subliminal desperation begins to accummulate. We are haunted by a sense of dread or simple *wrongness* about how things are. The more often we fail to make things ok, the stronger the sensations of despair will become.

I was so impressed with Tony's insight and the implications of our talk about it that I decided, playfully, to create a new syndrome: "Early Onset Extended Neural Hypervigilance Syndrome," or Richardson's Vigilance. My calling it this began playfully, but my experience since then has convinced me that this state of tension and unease is one that many people recognize in themselves and would gladly be free of.

The exercises that develop a tolerance for calm and a basis for letting well-being become ordinary are helpful in inviting the nervous sytem to re-structure itself and risk resting down.

BEGINNING TO LET THINGS BE OK

EXERCISE 67: Find a quiet place where you are unlikely to be startled or interrupted. Do your best to ensure this, e.g., lock the door, put up a sign, station a large dog outside. Sit in some way so that you are truly comfortable and your back can be upright. You can sit cross-legged or in *seiza* (on your heels like a martial artist) if those positions are genuinely comfortable for you. Otherwise, an armless, straight-backed chair with a cushion at your lower back is first-rate.

Just sit there, as simply as possible, without trying to do any-thing and without waiting for something to happen.

Very likely you will find it impossible. When you begin to feel uneasy, get up and walk around a bit, a few minutes maybe, before you sit down again. Do this four or five times. If you find yourself truly annoyed or agitated, stop and try the exercise again another day. Otherwise, let yourself notice, without worrying about it, all the things your mind comes up with to convince you that just sitting there quietly is either impossible or a bad idea. "This is stupid!" "I don't have *time* for this!" "This whole book is an insult to my intelligence!" "I have more important things to do with my time!" "Something awful will happen to me—or my chil-dren—if I'm not paying attention." "The dog will get out of the yard and get run over."

It's possible these announcements from your mind are based on a deeper feeling of unease or dread. See if you are willing to take the risk of sitting there without any agenda beyond just sitting for thirty sec-onds or so *just to see what will happen*. This may seem ludicrous but, believe me, it isn't. It is very likely that your body—stuck in time—does not actually believe that nothing bad will happen. Your body will tend to move, neurologically and neurochemically, into a waiting pos-ture—waiting for you to get over this mad idea and get back to worry and effort.

Trust the experiment enough to take that time and really notice when nothing bad happens. Take it in as real information, as deeply as you can, no matter how silly it may seem at first: "It's really true; I can sit quiet and easy for thirty seconds and get away with it."

Maybe you already have a tolerance for calm and well-being that is quite well-developed. Still, you might want to notice what your limits are. Give yourself ten minutes, or twenty, or an hour. Sometime you might want to give yourself a whole day. Remember, this is time with-out a task, in which you are not waiting for things to be different. (That includes not waiting for the time to be over, of course! If you find yourself waiting, rest down out of it, or give over the exercise for the time being.)

Over time, giving yourself this sort of opportunity will help your nervous system trust itself to rest down more, more often.

EXERCISE 68: As you sit without trying and without waiting, let your breath move so that it sounds a little like surf coming into shore on a calm sunny afternoon. Listen to the ocean sound of your breath and melt into the sound as fully as you can.

Time the exercise, as you did above, with respect for any uneasiness you may feel. Get up and walk when you want to, still melting into the ocean sound of your breath as fully as feels easy for you. Don't *make* yourself do any of these exercises. Take advantage of those times when you feel an actual attraction or interested willingness to try them out, see what they do.

After you have breathed in this way for as long as feels good to you, take a nap for five or ten minutes. Fall asleep if you can and will. If not, then move *towards* falling asleep without worrying about whether you get there or not.

EXERCISE 69: Sit in the same comfortable upright way and let your breath move again like the ocean. If you sigh from time to time, that will make variations in the surf sound and invite a deeper letting down. Choose something that reminds you of love—a flower, an object that you like to see, a photo of someone you love. Put it where you can easily see it as you sit. As your ears let you melt into the sound of your breath, let your eyes melt you into what you love. If you trust touch more than seeing, let yourself hold the object lovingly.

Go as deeply in the direction of feeling love presence as you feel safe to do in the moment. If the sense that things are basically ok arises, rest into it and let your cells drink it in. See if you can pause in the exercise before you feel startled or uneasy. It's best to take a nap while you are still feeling love presence.

Beyond Calm

When we have some experience that we can trust ease and calm as a base, we can begin to explore further. The temptation, I'm afraid, is to say, "Yum yum," and try to plunge into deeper pleasure states from a *base* of anger or fear or sadness. I have to tell you this will not work. (I tried, long and hard.) As one of my teachers said, it only leads to excitement and disappointment. States of bliss and ecstasy (for example) arise spontaneously from the ground of ease. It takes very little to invite them. But if we invite them from a base of un-ease, we enter into just another realm of struggle and defeat. The body will fight against "forgetting itself" until it feels calm and easy in current time. Until the raggy old Rent-a-Tigers of our past history are felt to have gone to their long reward, we will, as a body, refuse to surrender.

Do, please, begin each of these exercises with some time of resting down *for its own sake.* Ah, the sneakiness of our small mind! Calm and ease that we *make* in order to do other exercises is not the genuine article. Sigh. Begin again from the beginning. Isn't this infuriating? Manipulation and effort simply won't work. The gradual development of trust based on experience, and *allowing* the natural ground of ease to show itself, are the only ways into this playground.

On the other hand, ease and calm are progressive. We don't have to wait until we are perfect before playing with joy. What is one to do? Play. And get over onself. And play some more.

EXERCISE 70: Sit in the position you have found best in inviting ease and resting down. Rest down as well as you currently can. Trust the ease you know.

Sitting with your spine flexible and upright—something like the stem of a lily—rock gently from side to side. Rock slowly enough that you can enter into each moment of movement and awareness. Taste the qualities of sensation that arise as you move. Slowly let the range of your rocking get smaller and smaller until the outer movment of your body becomes invisible. Allow the inner movement to continue. Melt self into this inner movement. Let your breath change as it will to deepen the melting.

EXERCISE 71: In the same way, rock forward and back gently from your hip joints (not your back). Explore this new axis of movement, leaving your spine upright and flexible as you rock. Stay aware *in* and *as* the movement. Savor the sensations that arise. Gradually allow the arc of movement to lessen until visible movement disappears into inner movement. Surrender to that inner movmement. Melt awareness into it. Let breath and sound respond spontaneously to the sensations that arise with the inner movement and your union with it.

EXERCISE 72: Proceeding in this same way, let's have a go at putting your head on straight. First, move your head through the back-and-forth movement you use when you want to say "No." As before, let apparent movement disappear into inner movement. The more minute the final outer movements, the more inner movement will arise. Let breath loosen and sound arise.

Repeat with the up-and-down movement we use for "Yes" and then with the side-to-side movement that East Indians politely use to indicate they would like to be helpful, but... For each of these movements allow smaller and smaller outer movements to elicit and then dissolve into inner movements of fluid and energy. Rather than watch these inner flows, or talk to yourself about them, melt into and become one with them—always and only to the degree it feels happy and safe to do so.

If your habits of mind tell you you are hopeless and will never be able to let this flowing happen, this is a wonderful opportunity to be kind to yourself. Anyway, it isn't true. If *I* can learn to melt out of terror and suspicion into flow, then I take it for evident that, with time and patience and humor, anyone can.

This series of movements permits an inner "tune-up" which predisposes you, as a body, to move from ease into profound flow of energy and presence along and through the flow of your body. How much flow you are prepared to allow—*to be*—will vary a good deal from time to time but, as I say, if you persist with some patience and humor, your capacity to experience and to surrender to flow will certainly deepen and strengthen.

In describing the movement aspect of these exercises, I have not so far said much about the aspects of breath and sound. That is because the range of possibilities is endless. If your breath is long and slow, the flavor of sensation in the flow will be vastly different from if your breath is high and quick and makes choppy, rising waves in the flow. Equally, the sounds you make will "steer" the flow in many different directions of sensation and feeling. I invite you to play with your breath and the sounds you make while surrendered to flow. As one of my Tibetan teachers said to me on a memorable occasion, "Wouldn't you rather just see what happens?"

111

There is, however, one sound too important not to mention especially, and that is AH. AH is one of the three primary seed syllables, or formative sounds, adopted from Sanskrit by many tantricas, including the Tibetans. It is, among other things, the sound of surrender, the sound of release, the sound of interconnectedness, the sound of wonder. What follows is simply one way of exploring its depths. At any time of the day or night, AH is a blessing. The more fully it is integrated with movement and breath, the more fully it will touch you.

EXERCISE 73: Continuing to melt into the inner movement, let yourself voice the sound AH so that it flows through your whole body. Notice the many different qualities of AH, from relief to pleasure. Play with AH like a river of sound. Be the river. Allow yourself as much pleasure as feels safe and grateful to you.

While you are still in a state of pleasure or satisfaction, take a nap. As you move dozily in the direction of sleep, make little pleasure sounds with your lips. Luxuriate in the felt changes in the movements of fluid within your body. In particular, your fluids may feel pleasantly, sensuously, "slick" to you. This is what happy fluids feel like.

Ahem

Ok. So now we begin to know how to be angry freely, and how to come out of it with some ease and grace when it belongs to the past rather than the present. Ditto, we begin to know this with fear and sadness, and that begins to give us more emotional range and freedom of expression, less fear of feeling past feelings or present feelings.

Yeah, but what about real life? This is something people say when, in their hearts, they doubt that their social milieu will recognize or support the changes they are making in how they are. One aspect of "real life" that is particularly thorny for many is relationship. By which we usually mean only those relationships we have with people we live with, especially if we have sex with them. It's very true that, to integrate your new feelings and freedoms into your life, you will need to be willing to "be somebody else" with the people you are close to. That can create tension. Hell, it *does* create tension. After all, the person they went into relationship with was the one you were before!

Needless to say, it helps if you don't surprise them with a full-burn primate extravaganza the first time you are playing with anger. At least,

112

not without making an announcement first! If your partners, whether lovers or friends, have any interest at all, it is quite possible to change your milieu as you go by doing the exercises together.

If you want to try, you can have a lot of fun together. You can also, in time, free your relationships from much of their past luggage. There are two things I would like to suggest before you begin. One is to look at how to show up in the same spacetime together, whether for doing the exercises or some other purpose, and this we will look at in the next section. The other is what I call "safety brackets"—a clear understanding, which can only grow clearer with practice, that you are making a safe place for play and exploration—not "working on your relationship," which is frequently a deadly activity. That you will be present to each other, but each remains responsible for the emotional states he or she is making. That what happens in the safety bracket stays there and is not a weapon to be used later. That presence includes care and concern and is not a mask for avoidance.

Then you can let 'er rip. Go back and play all the games again, together. First, for safety reasons, let one person be angry or sad or scared at a time. Then trade. When you feel more confidence and flexibility, you can both rev up at the same time. It's good to have, as part of the safety bracket, an understanding that either partner can stop the game at any time.

When you find that you are no longer afraid of what you feel, no longer even afraid of being afraid, no longer afraid that you might do harm when you are angry, then (and only from true fearlessness on both sides), you can play with one person making anger and the other making fear or sadness. Then trade. Always trade, to keep things balanced. Nobody wants to be bad guy or underdog all the time.

So now, before playing, we need actually to meet each other.

Let's Get This Turkey in the Air

The turkey of human relationships is this: most of us are waiting—and waiting—and waiting—to be reassured that the relationship in question will end in a couple of hours at 4 a.m. *or* that it will continue deathlessly till the end of time. If only we could agree on what creates safety! Usually, though, one person in this polarity is waiting for one reassurance and the other, for the other. What we seem quite sure of, however, is that until some conditions are met, surrender to *mutual* flow isn't in the cards.

It doesn't take a genius to figure out that these conditions recede endlessly into the distance. Even if they appear to be met, they are always subject to change. *We* are subject to change! So while we are waiting to fulfill them and stabilize them and renew them and nail them down and otherwise get it right for ourselves, a lot of water can go under the bridge.

The ironic, when not openly caustic, remarks that men make about women and women make about men (or men about men and women about women, come to that) reflect the on-going, apparently interminable, frustration most of us feel because we are rarely ever mutually present to each other, as free of conditions as possible.

In this section, we are going to look at some of the simple ways you and a partner can, if you should want to, "show up" in the same space and time with each other and actually *meet*. Having met, you may then feel inclined to spend more time with each other, doing something together in communion, whether it be making love (for one day or a thousand—oops, here we go again!) or building bridges.

What do I mean by "mutual"? I mean the willingness and the capacity to notice (and continue to notice) that you *are* and to notice at the same time that someone else *is*. To notice your own reality and presence without losing the other; to notice the reality and presence of the other without losing yourself.

Usually, we ping pong back and forth from "I'm real and you're not" to "You're real and I'm not" in whatever relationships we are in. This is how we manage so persistently to miss each other. In some relationships, we are the "real" one most of the time; in others, we lose ourselves most of the time and the other is more real to us than we are.

To learn to be mutually present in more and more of our relationships—whether the other person has learned how or not—is a blessing that never wears out and never grows old.

Maybe you would prefer to begin learning what it is to be mutual with another being by practicing first with some creature less problematical than a human being. That's fine. Pick any being you fancy: a cat, a goldfish, a petunia. They don't even have to be physically present if you can feel their reality without. Just check yourself first for a true willingness to meet this being without distance or disguise.

114

EXERCISE 74: Sit comfortably with the being you have chosen to practice with. Close your eyes. (If you are both human beings and both doing the exercise, both of you follow the instructions at the same time.) Turn your attention to all the information that tells you that you *are*. There is an amazing amount of it, really. Even with your eyes closed, there may be pictures in your mind. Or words you hear. Or sounds. Bring your attention closer and closer to perception itself—not so much *what* is perceived but that perceiving is happening. You will encounter all the signals your body puts out to tell you that it is *there*—you-as-a-body are there—as well as where you are and what position you are in. There will also be those signals that arise from movements of energy and presence. Many many of these signals give you information about *how* you are. Take in this information. Do not be too much distracted by the *how*, but continue on to the core information *that* you are. Presence itself.[3]

When you are resting aware in presence, even if it seems to you little, open your eyes and look at your partner. Notice that this other being—whether human or fish, cat or petunia—also *is*. This being has the same reality and presence as you do. You have the same reality and presence they do.

If you begin to lose awareness of yourself in noticing the reality of the other, close your eyes again and recollect all the signs and signals of your being. When you feel again a bit steady, open your eyes and begin again.

Often when we begin to move towards mutual presence and awareness, we have to move attention back and forth—which is what we usually do, anyway—but with more clarity about what we are doing with our attention and the effects it has. First aware of oneself. Then aware of the other. Aware of oneself. Aware of the other. Back and forth. After some time of riding this swing, your attention will relax and spread to include you both. There you are, mutual. If your mind flickers and tightens, just back off, rest, and begin again. Take a short, dozy nap before you begin again. It takes a special set of mind muscles to pull this off and, like everything new, it takes patience.[4]

When you come to mutuality, you will find a number of positive states spontaneously arising: gladness at the being of the other, a wish that they be well and happy, delight in *being* together, and an inner quietude about being altogether. These are not "made" states in the sense that anger, fear, or sadness may be made by habit or intention, but are the underlying basic qualities of relaxed being and presence. As these states arise for you, let them be visible and audible to your partner. Notice that sharing them, deepens them.

In the beginning, you may not be able to remain mutual for very long. Keep in mind that mutuality is a markedly mature capacity. It takes nurturing and strengthening. When in doubt whether to worry or be kind, be kind.

Remember to rest before you are tired or go flat in the exercise. Nap, so that your body can incorporate the learning you have invited by doing the exercise.

All the exercises for inducing calm and flow can be done mutually with great pleasure and benefit.

Honey in the Void

If you and your partner will sit quietly—or bawdily—together and re-trace the path of experience from tolerance for calm through beginning to let things be ok to going beyond calm...if you will do this from a position of mutual presence and awareness...if you will do this persistently and playfully, with humor and a willingness to see what happens, then a great mystery will open to you: you will discover an experience that best goes into English as "openness" or "spaciousness." You will discover that when awareness rests in openness, vastness becomes sweet.

Like the rabbit gazing wordlessly at the moon, I point you towards that sphere of experience called "honey in the void." More I won't say; a whole lifetime is barely enough to explore it. But I wish you and your partner the willingness to discover it together with love and gladness and compassion. May your heart expand into space and fill all experience with love.

Bon Voyage

I am going to say good-bye now. Many people, a surprising number, have written over the last ten years to say they have found *The Lover Within* very helpful in their lives. That is good news. I hope this new incarnation will prove even more interesting and exciting and helpful than the last. I thank you all for reading the book and, especially, for trying out the exercises, which is what makes all the difference.

I wish you entirely well and happy.

Notes

1. My gratitude, not only to George, but to Bob and Mary Goulding, the originators of this very effective combination of Gestalt Therapy and Transactional Analysis.

2. The expression "to rest down" came into English from one of my Tibetan teachers, Vairocana Tulku Rinpoche.

3. If you happen to be feeling annihilated on a particular day, notice that the sensations of annihilation, however obnoxious, are very vivid indeed. In this case, also, go past the *how* you are (in this case, self-annihilated) to *that* you are (which remains true, though temporarily painful).

4. The thing about naps, briefly, is this: When we encounter a challenge—and learning anything new is always a challenge—our whole bodily being revs up to meet it. Ok, well and good, but if we don't let down afterwards, we don't actually *learn* from meeting the challenge. It remains for body and mind an instance of distress. You will find the long version of this, and the scientific supports, in Hans Seyle's works on stress and distress and how they are different. Our habit is to turn stress into distress, which is one of the things these exercises work to undermine.

16
Responses to *The Lover Within*

A wealth of practical exercises, a gem for spiritual practitioners, a handbook for mind/body devotees, and a must for all of us who simply want more aliveness.

The Lover Within explores energetic boundaries in an easy, practical and enlivening way. Doing the exercises works; experiencing them has brought me the discovery of both myself and others and has transformed my attitudes and expectations in all my personal relationships.
Karen Bell, Director, Somatics Australia

The ease with which *The Lover Within* moves from the written word to instructions for the simple and extremely effective practices makes this book a real treasure.

Kerrie Tooth

Julie Henderson, with delightful sparklings of whimsy and playfulness, tells us clearly that the business of making friends with ourselves and becoming more fully incarnate doesn't have to be so serious and difficult after all! A deliciously subversive map for those helping themselves and others on the path to self-liberation.
Llewellyn Wishart, Melbourne

In my experience, personal growth has always been hard work. Julie has since shown me in an effortless and, dare I say, simple way that feeling good can become an ordinary state,—no matter how hard I try to make it.
Mark Breadner, Yoga teacher and Somatic Therapist

This woman is a genius.
Carlie Hindhaugh, 12 year old workshop attender

Thank you for sending a copy of your wonderful, easy-to-read, and most helpful fun book. What a great book this is!

I enjoyed your course immensely and I plan to come to the one year training you are offering.

Daniel Süsstrunk, Munich, Germany

I have learned many things in my 4 years training to be a therapist, but the most valuable practical and grounding work I have done has been with Julie Henderson.

Vas Alvanos, Sydney, Australia

I have had the blessing of studying with Julie Henderson in person for a year and a half. At various points during that time I'd pick up *The Lover Within* and try the first exercise. After months of sporadic "practice" I was able to notice how much I compress my energy in my pelvis while being "sexual." "Feel touched in the biggest space possible," said Julie. Just being able to notice the compression has enabled me to change the habit.

Rabia Mead, San Francisco, California

Julie's exercises and teaching have given me riches and satisfaction that I previously could not even imagine I deserved. The riches are now in my relationships, work and family life and have added depth to all these areas. Best of all, I just feel better and enjoy more.

Peter Tooth, Businessman, Therapist, and Yoga teacher

I started working with Julie Henderson while going to graduate school, at the recommendation of a Buddhist scholar. I read *The Lover Within* and then sought her out. She is now on the very short list of people I really respect.

Her work was like a lab session for the classes in Buddhism I was taking. She would say, "Nothing stands still: feel this pulsation." Or, "'Emptiness'? I stay a mile upstream of that word; I prefer 'openness.' Feel this." And then, somehow, she would induce an experience that showed how the world is not cramped and crowded, but open and full of possibilities.

She is so capable, in part because of an extremely wide education: she is familiar with everything from theater to quantum physics. She doesn't flash her knowledge around, but she has it. She has intellectual as well as practical depth. It is thanks to Julie that I am surviving my stressful life. My body feels twice as awake as it did before I met her, and happier too. And she gave me, with *The Lover Within*, a way to work with energy. A magic lady, she.

Birrell Walsh, Contributing Editor, MicroTimes Magazine

The Lover Within is an extroardinary book because it gives us a simple language for dealing with a subtle, familiar dimension of ordinary experience: our felt experience of presence in space. In the West we have no language for this; learning the language of *The Lover Within* through its series of structured exercises brings choices that are largely unconscioius into focus, opening ways to relaxation and pleasure.

The Lover Within stretches beyond traditional Buddhist teaching because it takes an egalatarian approach to "esoteric" experiences. It articulates "energetic" aspects of embodiment in language and exercises that are accessible to an uninitiated Western audience. By doing this (as I see it, though I am not an expert) it provides a new context for critiquing the traditions, a context, for example, in which assertions about how we experience our embodiment can be tested. I recall, in a workshop lead by Julie, creating energetic pathways that diverged wildly from those familiar in acupuncture, for instance. At the same time it provides an excellent corrective to Western accounts of sexuality that focus on the physical and emotional without being sensitive to how we really live our contact with each other: how we "touch" each other (or choose not to) in the subtle ways that go with feeling we are or are not "one flesh" with our partners.

Here's an example of how, concretely, the work described in *The Lover Within* helps me in everyday contexts: When I notice myself feeling uncomfortably "contracted" (withdrawn, in fear, from my surroundings—something one can do with one's "sense" of being present in a space largely independently of how much space one occupies physically!), I recall the lessons of *The Lover Within* and "feather" my presence (inducing very fine pulsations); or contract inwards tightly and release and expand out; or increase the "density" of my sense of presence, sharpening my sense of the boundary between me and my surroundings, so that I feel more protected; or pulsate quite robustly (contracting in and expanding out across some comfortable range); or expand out and fill a space with my presence ... In different circumstances each of these, and sometimes a series of actions like this, becomes a pathway towards a more relaxed, centred way of being. This among other things I find professionally useful. I facilitate better, when I'm leading multi-party, multi-disciplinary workshops on environmental management problems, for example. And I deal more effectively with anxiety generally. The skills to do this would have been inaccessible without *The Lover Within* —or something similar (and I know of no book that comes close to *The Lover Within* for its elegant simplicity in this area).

Greg Walkerden, Environmental manager/
environmental conflict resolution facilitator

Dear Julie:

You have changed my life with your book. I have known I must really have changed since the day I met my ex-husband on the street and he asked me, "When is Julie Henderson giving her next course? You have changed in such a good way since reading her book and taking courses from her. I would like to experience that too."

Yesterday I had a long phone conversation with my mother. We talked about what an extraordinary year this has been. My little company is flourishing, and the prospects for next year are even better. My au pair girl has just written me a moving letter. She is leaving after two years here. She writes how grateful she is for my support and trust.

In the spring I met my dream man. Since then we have moved in together, and he said recently, "I am so glad that I found you—how tedious to be stuck with an ordinary woman."

I know that all this has a great deal to do with you. I have shifted from a space of trouble and worry into a space where anything is possible. You showed me that space and led me into it. My thanks to you, Julie.

Dr. Agnes Kunkel

Appendix A

The Short Course

To experience satisfying sexual union with yourself or with a partner, you need:
    —high charge (relative to your normal base line)
    —a relaxed, toned, flexible system capable of
        containment
        pulsation
        reflexive re-distribution of energy
    —contact (whether physical, emotional, energetic, or spiritual) that allows you to feel touched
        by self
        with another
        with/by life

Why:
    —High charge in a *rigid* system creates displeasure. The person will either avoid touch *or* move towards rapid, frequent release.
    —Low charge (usually in a contracted or collapsed energetic system) means that the systemic energy never reaches the point of reflexive release.
    —Lacking the kind(s) of contact you value, touch will feel flat, mechanical, or hollow; so will sex. And life.

The more toned and flexible you are energetically and muscularly, emotionally and mentally, the more charge and the more life you can contain and the more pleasure you can experience. This is true of your being at all, as well as in the release and re-distribution of "extra" energy in sex (and other experiences of union).

Appendix B

The Inner Courtship

My own experience of the progression of this process of energetic "courtship" goes this way:

1. First, energy is flowing around us more than through us (because of the quality of the boundaries we have made). Energy within the boundaries is more in stasis than in movement. Also we are not very conscious of this life energy, inside or outside. *Many* people are subliminally aware of energy currents, exchanges, and flavours and rely very heavily on these perceptions. Usually they don't reveal that they do, through lack of either vocabulary or validation for their perceptions. Such things are "not talked about"—until someone talks about them.

2. Then, given an opportunity through exercises or other guidance, energy begins to flow in the body in certain limited areas, the first that are willing to open. There is visible vibration, often quite jerky. Sometimes the person feels nervous about this "loss of control" or "weakness".

3. Gradually, as more areas open, energy moves through the whole body but tends to remain large-scale and near the surface. During this same period, the vibration and trembling begin to get finer. This is the beginning of that "higher frequency vibration" all of those esoteric manuals talk about.

4. Gradually the vibration reaches fineness throughout the body (or most of it) and begins to touch deeper tissues.

5. Vibration becomes flow.

6. Pulsation begins to arise.

7. The pulsation becomes finer and finer and reaches deeper and deeper into the tissues of the body until it touches and re-enlivens individual cells. This is the luminous life of childhood. This time we are conscious; indeed the cells are conscious. Being is conscious.

8. The energy of this cellular pulsation radiates as light. We experience the energy of life directly, as both personal and nonpersonal.

124

Appendix C

Advanced Exercises

In pursuing this work on your own or with someone else, tremendous honesty and courage are necessary. You need to know—to be willing to know—what you want, not just what you "want to want" or think you ought to want. Also, if you separate your "consciousness" from your bodily being and try to *make* your body do what "you" want when "it" wants something else, nothing of any value will arise. (The *I Ching* refers to this kind of struggle when it says that even if you win a prize three times in one day, you will have lost it before the sun goes down.) Creating a cooperative union of your consciousness and body leads inevitably to deepening pleasure and harmony in being. You will have felt some of this movement practising the exercises in this book. This final appendix includes a few relatively advanced exercises that you may enjoy. I hope you find that you are beginning to create your own.

EXERCISE 75: Produce a happy feeling by expanding and pulsating or an expansive pulsation through feeling happy. (Use a memory, create a current situation, or expand voluntarily.) Allow the energy of your expansion to retain this flavour of happiness and walk with it into the world. Allow this "flavour" of energy to touch your environment. Notice the effects.

EXERCISE 76: Find a safe, quiet place. Sit or lie quietly. "Intend" orgasmic pleasure. Allow your response to this intention. Setting aside the strangeness of simply "intending" such a thing, notice where in your body you deny consent to this response. Don't worry yourself over this lack of consent; one of the strongest nonverbal messages you ever received probably has to do with the "impossibility" of this.

(How do you learn to walk? You see it done; you imagine it, probably without knowing that you do. There is kinesthetic resonance from the seeing to proprioceptive cells throughout your body. There is then an impulse to movement, which you practise until the neural pathways are steady and strong. As Erickson said often, at least half of learning to walk is sitting down.)

So. Visualise yourself in ecstatic response. Relax into sounds of pleasure. As you do so, merge your awareness with the visualisation and sound, and allow your body to respond kinesthetically to the intention of orgasm. Enjoy the pleasure that arises, and surrender further. Continue this positive feedback loop until you reach a limit or are satisfied.

EXERCISE 77: Improvise a song (preferably with lyrics) expressing what you feel. Surrender to the movement of sound and feeling. Notice how your experience of being changes.

EXERCISE 78: Find a quiet place on the shore of a bay or lake where the waves are gentle (gentle!). Lie down on your back parallel to the water. Place yourself right on the line where the waves break, so that sometimes the waves come almost to you, sometimes you are lightly touched by them, and sometimes they surround you. (Be conservative, at least to begin with.) As you pick your spot and lie down, notice your attitude. How do you feel about what is about to happen? Can you relax? Can you close your eyes? (And relax?) How do you feel about this level of uncertainty and vulnerability? Practise surrender to the uncertainty of how you will be touched.

This exercise will give you immediate insight into how you feel about trust, touch, and the uncertainties inherent in being alive. Be respectful of your limits. Sound your response. Consider singing your responses.

A Note on the Structure of the Lover Within

The Lover Within is balanced between formal and friendly intentions, and its structure reflects that. Formal structure is based on an Ericksonian model of layered and partially indirect access to information. The first, and most obvious, layer of content concerns the energetic aspects of sexuality, relationship, and union. The second level of information is discussed overtly in part and by implication throughout. This level is concerned with voluntary energy distribution, with the relationship of energy distribution in the body to feeling and behaviour, and with how to gain some measure of choice over how one feels. The third level of information focusses on inducing (in the Ericksonian sense) the specific sensations of *being*, as contrasted with *existing*. This distinction in the quality of consciousness is something that can be better taught by demonstration and induction than explained; for that reason, this third layer relies almost entirely on nonlinear communication.

The topic of sexuality, sexual intimacy, and other possibilities of union acts as a kind of "grabber", attracting and focussing conscious attention and making energy available for the other levels of learning. The second layer is most clearly visible in the chapters on "Energetic Habits" and "The Energetic Breaths", which formulate an approach to character and structure in the energy body. The third layer proceeds by instruction in the skills of direct perception of life energy and of voluntary distribution of personal energies—in daily life as well as in sexual relationship. These skills are then applied to volitional merging and separation of energy fields between partners, the voluntary creation of energetic dipole and charge, and the experience of a variety of patterns of energetic union.

The book has the more obvious form of a conversation with the reader. This conversation is relatively informal and ranges over a wide variety of apparent (and actual) topics, e.g., the sources of sexual misery and sexual pleasure; life energy, generally and sexually; human boundaries in the context of quantum mechanics; how our energetic boundaries and energy level affect our relationships; our "energetic habits"; what to do about our boundaries and habits; how to begin to relate to life as a potentially pleasurable "love affair" rather than a bed of pain. Dispersed throughout this conversation are sixty-three exercises—a kind of programmed learning series—in how to experience life energy directly, how to move it voluntarily and with purpose, to increase freedom and pleasure in being, and to increase the individual's (or couple's) capacity for charge, excitement, pleasure, and intimacy with or without sexual intercourse.

The theoretical and experiential bases of the book are drawn from such usually disparate fields as bioenergetics and somatics, acting training, meditation, Ericksonian hypnotherapy, martial arts, and quantum theory. The tone, however, is friendly and practical, so that the reader should find it possible with some ease to experience results of increased liveliness, pleasure, and freedom of choice.

In relation to other disciplines, *The Lover Within* offers certain particular possible contributions. In a transpersonal context, it represents a "re-invention" of the energetic aspects of tantra. From a bioenergetic or somatic point of view, its main interest is perhaps as an alternative discussion of boundary issues and an energetic approach to character structure. For sexologists and sex therapists, it introduces the concept of charge as a factor in sexual desire, excitement, and pleasure, and offers some effective means for working directly with charge in treatment.

Appendix E

Appropriate Touch

Virtually everyone now living in the western world has been touch deprived from birth. I know that is a very big thing to say. It is also a terrible thing, and it's true.

We were born, which is a stressful bit of business in itself. Then for most of us, instead of being allowed to lie naked on the naked bosom of our mother, reconnecting to her heart and rhythms, allowing breath to come naturally and spontaneously, allowing the umbilical cord to finish its job, giving the placenta time to be born and all of its rich nutrients and blood to drain into our tiny new body—instead of this, what? Held upside down and swatted into a gasping first breath, cord cut while it still holds the pulse of life (and so cutting us abruptly off from what has been our connection to source), loss of one-third of our blood supply still in the placenta, wrapped up in cloth that cuts us off from contact and from our main source of information about where we are and how we are—so that, even if we are with our mother and everything is ok, we can't know that—and, in fact, usually taken away even from that muffled information that we are where we should be and, instead, left in a void of disconnection.

Great, eh? Then things begin to get complicated. The skin is our largest organ. We keep it covered up so that the information it can give us is limited to the textures of cloth. We are gradually taught to touch skin to skin only with our hands—sometimes with parts of our faces— except in sexual situations. This creates a great ignorance and deprivation, frustration and resentment in us.

Every body needs to be touched. Every body of us needs to be touched—appropriately—as part of everyday life—like good food— what we like, when we need it—so it isn't such a big deal. So we don't feel like we are starving to death in some mysterious way we can hardly identify.

Most of us don't have appropriate touch in our lives—touch that is a gift, not a demand; touch that we invite or wish for, not that we put up with. Touch that is *right* for us. Right for *us*. In time and place, quality and quantity.

No doubt in some nature video you have seen troops of chimpanzee or gorillas sitting around together in two's or three's, lying together in comfortable heaps, playing and grooming each other. As beings with bodies—beings who are, after all, genetically primates—it is something like this that we need—ordinary, everyday, satisfying.

But, you may say, I'm not an ape—I'm a human being—I'm *civilized*! Too true. But a huge proportion of your brain is designed to receive the signals of this sort of ordinary, playful, uncontaminated touching as the sign that things are well with you—and to release the appropriate "Mmmmmm. Yum. Yum." neurochemistry.

If we are truly fortunate, we have managed to create for ourselves a circumstance in which touching is warm, free, uncomplicated, and full of mutual presence. Sometimes sexual and ecstatic, more often not.

If, like most, we have not managed this, or if our history, like many, has created confusion about when and if and what kind of touching is ok, we may feel bewilderment or ignorance or resentment about any sort of touching altogether. Or wonder if there is such a thing as appropriate touching. We may need to re-learn to recognize when and how and what kind—and if—touching is the right thing for us right now.

Bibliography

Alexander, Gerda. *Eutony: The Holistic Discovery of the Total Person.* New York: Felix Morrow, 1986.

This is an introduction to the profound work developed by Alexander over the last 55 years. Her work is not only a method of healing and treatment but also a Western meditation on *being* through the body. Emphasis on proprioceptive perception of body spaces, movement of energy (by intention and focus of attention), development of contactfulness and presence, voluntary modification of physical tonus.

Andersen, Marianne S., and Savary, Louis M. *Passages: A Guide for Pilgrims of the Mind.* New York: Harper and Row, 1972.

Guided, timed exercises with specific goals and intentions for the alteration of consciousness.

Baker, Elsworth F., M.D. *Man in the Trap: The Causes of Blocked Sexual Energy.* New York: Macmillan, 1967.

A discussion of character structure in vivid psychoanalytic jargon. Whether it is helpful or a laugh depends on the languages you speak.

Barker, Clive. *Theatre Games.* London: Methuen, 1977.

Physical, social, emotional games that make for more powerful, expressive, flexible actors—and do the same for other interested people.

Benjamin, Benjamin E. *Are You Tense? The Benjamin System of Muscular Therapy.* New York: Pantheon, 1978.

A system of deep massage and muscular therapy, as it says. If you are interested, study four or five dissimilar systems; then create your own to suit. This system includes a "Tension Test" to check yourself out.

Bertherat, Thérèse, and Bernstein, Carol. *The Body Has Its Reasons: Anti-exercises and Self-awareness.* New York: Avon, 1979. (First published in France, 1976.)

Like Alexander and Gorman, Bertherat has discovered that, in exercise and in movement, less is often more.

Briggs, John P., Ph.D., and Peat, F. David, Ph.D., *Looking Glass Universe: The Emerging Science of Wholeness.* Simon & Schuster, New York: 1984.

This book didn't come out until after I wrote *The Lover Within,* but I include it in the bibliography because it is an absolutely first rate introduction to the thought of Bohm, Pribram, Prigogine, & Sheldrake. An exciting intellectual roller coaster ride into the "new" science.

Bubba Free John. *Love of the Two-Armed Form: The Free and Regenerative Function of Sexuality in Ordinary Life, and the Transcendance of Sexuality in True Religious or Spiritual Practice.*
Middletown, California: Dawn Horse Press, 1978.

This is a *very* advanced text. Robyn Speyer showed it to me after I had already written *The Lover Within.* I would suggest you wait until you have a direct experience of what Bubba Free John calls "the Blissful Current of Life-Energy" (p. 15) before taking it on. You need also to be willing to deal with a fairly specialised vocabulary in which the variations from normal usage are not always obvious. Nevertheless, if you want to reach for the highest peach on the tree, this is a good book to have.

Capra, Fritjov. *The Tao of Physics.* (2nd ed.) Boulder, Colorado: Shambhala, 1983.
Relates Eastern and Western views of reality in the light of quantum physics.

Castaneda, Carlos. *Teachings of Don Juan: A Yaqui Way of Knowledge.* New York: Washington Square Press, 1968.

Chekhov, Michael. *To the Actor on the Techniques of Acting.* New York: Harper and Row, 1953.
A brilliant work with very simple, effective exercises using body posture to influence emotion and energy distribution.

Douglas, Nik, and Slinger, Penny. *Sexual Secrets.* New York: Destiny Books, 1979.
Encyclopedic, coffee-table sort of book on tantra. Lots of pictures.

Dowman, Keith, trans. *Sky Dancer: The Secret Life and Songs of the Lady Yeshe Tsogyel.* London: Routledge and Kegan Paul, 1984.
This is an alternative translation of the same text as *Mother of Knowledge.* The book includes learned essays.

Dowman, Keith, trans. *The Divine Madman: The Sublime Life and Songs of Drukpa Kunley.* Clearlake, California: Dawn Horse Press, 1980.
A "secret" life from the vajrayana tradition, i.e., it includes references to sexuality as a part of the road to awakening. It doesn't talk about how it works; that's up to Drukpa Kunley. We should all be so lucky as to meet him somewhere.

Downing, George. *The Massage Book.* New York: Random House, 1972.
Introduction to Esalen-style massage by one of its designers.

Erickson, Milton H., M.D. *The Collected Papers of Milton H. Erickson on Hypnosis, vols. I–IV.* Ernest L. Rossi, ed. New York: Irvington Publishers, 1980.
Erickson in all flavours.

Erickson, Milton H., M.D., and Rossi, Ernest L., Ph.D. *Experiencing Hypnosis: Therapeutic Approaches to Altered States.* New York: Irvington Publishers, 1981.
As with everything of which Erickson was author or co-author, the best approach is to read it once trying to put together all the "too much" information linearly until your brain fogs, and then read it again without trying. Is it more important to know—or to know that you know? The older Erickson is never communicating *only* what he seems to be communicating. Get out of his way as much as you can and let him teach you.

Erickson, Milton H., Rossi, Ernest L. *Hypnotherapy: An Exploratory Casebook.* New York: Irvington Publishers, 1979.
Another introduction to how to alter consciousness for healing that is both more and less than itself depending on your own state of consciousness while reading it.

Erickson, Milton H., Rossi, Ernest L., and Rossi, Sheila I. *Hypnotic Realities: The Induction of Clinical Hypnosis and Forms of Indirect Suggestion.* New York: Irvington Publishers, 1976.
Erickson teaching induction by doing it. His remarks on himself are lovely and often full of hidden humour.

Feldenkrais, Moshe. *Awareness Through Movement.* New York: Harper and Row, 1972.
Exercises (in my terms) to learn how to let the body talk to the body and to let the body re-educate itself.

Gendlin, Eugene T., Ph.D. *Focusing.* New York: Everest House, 1978.
An entire book devoted to noticing proprioceptive effects of communication from "body" to "mind" and back.

Geba, Dr. Bruno Hans. *Breathe Away Your Tension.* New York: Random House, 1973.
Combines deep breathing and autosuggestion to influence energy flow and states of mind.

Gorman, David. *The Body Moveable. Blueprints of the Human Musculo-skeletal System: Its Structure, Mechanics, Locomotor and Postural Functions, Vols. I-III.* Vancouver, B.C.: Kromonium Productions, 1981.
This is my favourite anatomy book. Gorman has great humour and tenacity and even greater insight into intention, consent, and freedom of movement.

Guenther, Herbert V. *Tibetan Buddhism in Western Perspective.* Emeryville, California: Dharma Publishing, 1977.
This is a scholar's book; they don't come any better than Guenther, but you really have to want to read it.

Gunther, Bernard. *Energy Ecstasy and Your Seven Vital Chakras.* (2nd ed.) Los Angeles: The Guild of Tutors Press, 1979.
Visualisation, breath, and sound for moving energy and as the basis for meditation.

Gunther, Bernard. *Sense Relaxation: Below Your Mind.* New York: Collier Books, 1968.
A classic introduction to enlivenment of and through the body. Exercises and hints on touching.

Gyatso, Geshe Kelsang. *Clear Light of Bliss: Mahamudra in Vajrayana Buddhism.* London: Wisdom Publications, 1982.
One of the very most advanced of all spiritual tantras. If you are convinced you know what's real, try this. Lovely to discover that, of the three categories of beings capable of achieving enlightenment, human beings have the best chance. A very advanced practice from a world view in which energetic realities are perhaps more fully incorporated than they are anywhere else.

Hanna, Thomas. *The Body of Life.* New York: Alfred A. Knopf, 1980.
An introduction to the "soma"—the body alive and moving in space and time. Tom Hanna trained with Feldenkrais and, I think, has gone beyond his teacher.

Heckler, Richard Strozzi. *The Anatomy of Change: East/West*

Approaches to Body/Mind Therapy. Boulder, Colorado: Shambhala, 1984.

Heckler, Richard Kent. *The Body/Mind Interface.* San Francisco: Freeperson Press, 1975.
An interesting collection of essays on the body/mind marriage. Heckler teaches at the Lomi School and heads an aikido dojo.

Hessel, Sidi. *The Articulate Body.* New York: St. Martin's Press, 1978.
Exercises specifically to release and realign joints. Since many interruptions of energy flow occur at joints, these exercises can be very helpful if you have a specific joint in mind.

Houston, F. M., D.C. *The Healing Benefits of Acupressure.* New Canaan, Connecticut: Keats Publishing, 1974.
Very clear visual presentation of the location of pressure points and some remarks on what they influence. Knowledge of these points can increase the effectiveness of your touching. I recommend you practise on yourself and see if you agree with the observations of this (or any other) author on the effects of pressure on these points.

Houston, Jean. *The Possible Human: A Course in Extending Your Physical, Mental, and Creative Abilities.* Los Angeles: J. P. Tarcher, 1982.
An extension of her earlier work (with Robert Masters) exploring mind and body. Emphasis here on integration and expansion of faculties.

Hover, Robert Harry. *How to Direct the Life Force to Dispel Mild Aches and Pains.* La Mirada, California: The Hover Company, 1979.
Taking an entirely practical and pragmatic approach, Hover deals with such practices as inner vision and the energetic constructs associated with discomfort and illness: how to see them and how to remove them. The techniques derive from the author's lengthy experience of vipassana meditation.

Ichazo, Oscar. *Arica Psychocalisthenics.* New York: Simon and Schuster, 1976.
Ichazo's basic system of movement meditation for psycho-physical integration, alteration of mood, and so on.

Jung, C. G. *Mysterium Coniunctionis: An Inquiry into the Separation and Synthesis of Psychic Opposites in Alchemy.* Trans. by R. .F. C. Hull. Bollingen Series XX. New York: Bollingen Foundation, 1963.
This monumental work, often regarded as monumentally obscure, makes a lot more sense if regarded from the perspective of energetic movement towards union—intrapersonal, interpersonal, transpersonal.

Kaplan, Helen Singer, M.D., Ph.D. *The New Sex Therapy: Active Treatment of Sexual Dysfunctions.* New York: Brunner/Mazel, 1974.
A very condensed and competent presentation of the medical/behavioural approach to sexuality and sex therapy. (It was the failure of this approach to identify or relieve my own frustrations that prompted me to re-examine my direct experience and which led finally to a vocabulary of experience that made sense of what I felt and wanted.) I approve of this book though it suffers conceptually (in my

view) from the lack of such concepts as *charge*.

Kaplan, Helen Singer, M.D., Ph.D. *The New Sex Therapy, Vol. II: Disorders of Sexual Desire and Other New Concepts and Techniques in Sex Therapy*. New York: Brunner/Mazel, 1979.

The first discussion (I know of) of desire as a focus of sex therapy. "With some exceptions ISD [inhibited sexual desire] patients . . . have a relatively poor prognosis with all treatment methods currently employed." (p. 56) Energetic and bioenergetic approaches, of course, are outside her view and so are not considered.

Keleman, Stanley. *In Defense of Heterosexuality*. Berkeley, California: Center Press, 1982.

Right now, Keleman and Boadella are the most exciting theoreticians of the relationship between experience, development, and somatic structures that I know of.

Keleman, Stanley. *Somatic Reality: Bodily Experience and Emotional Truth*. Berkeley, California: Center Press, 1979.

Keleman, Stanley. *The Human Ground: Sexuality, Self and Survival*. (Revised and expanded ed.) Palo Alto, California: Science and Behavior Books, 1975.

Keleman, Stanley. *Your Body Speaks Its Mind*. Berkeley, California: Center Press, 1975.

Kent, Caron. *The Puzzled Body: A New Approach to the Unconscious*. London: Vision Press, 1969.

A very interesting book by a mainstream psychotherapist who let himself notice the physical changes in the body that take place as part of (chicken following egg following chicken) psychological change and growth.

Khanna, Madhu. *Yantra: The Tantric Symbol of Cosmic Unity*. London: Thames and London, 1979.

A book flourishing with illustrations, the images that have arisen in the tantric tradition investigating the movement of union with life.

Krieger, Dolores, Ph.D., R.N. *The Therapeutic Touch: How To Use Your Hands to Help or To Heal*. Englewood Cliffs, New Jersey: Prentice-Hall, 1979.

A fine introduction to perception and direction of energy for healing. Helpful anecdotes and exercises.

Kurtz, Ron, and Prestera, Hector, M.D. *The Body Reveals*. San Francisco: Harper and Row, 1976.

The best introduction there is to reading the structural language of the body. Lots of pictures and silhouettes that help to see experience in the body.

LeBoyer, Frederick. *Loving Hands: The Traditional Indian Art of Baby Massage*. New York: Alfred A. Knopf, 1976.

Great pictures of a great principle in action: loving touching grounds us lovingly in the flesh. A lifelong gift for any baby or for healing touch of anyone feeling small.

Leonard, George. *The End of Sex: Erotic Love After the Sexual Revolution*. Los Angeles: J. P. Tarcher, 1983.

A popular look at the effects on people of separating "sex" from life and intimacy. It calls for a renewed appreciation of the erotic.

LeShan, Lawrence. *Alternate Realities.* New York: Balantine Books, 1977.
A speculation on our capacity to alter the "rules" that make Reality real.

LeShan, Lawrence. *The Medium, The Mystic, and the Physicist.* New York: Viking Press, 1974.

LeShan, Lawrence, and Margenau, Henry. *Einstein's Space and Van Gogh's Sky: Physical Reality and Beyond.* New York: Macmillan, 1982.
An expansion of the earlier book on alternate realities in collaboration with the physicist who catalysed it.

Lowen, Alexander, M.D. *The Betrayal of the Body.* New York: Macmillan, 1967.

Lowen, Alexander, M.D. *Bioenergetics.* New York: Coward, McCann and Geoghagan, 1975.
The fullest single exposition of Lowen's system of developmental character structures revealed in physical structure.

Lowen, Alexander, M.D. *Depression and the Body: The Biological Basis of Faith and Reality.* New York: Penguin, 1972.

Lowen, Alexander, M.D. *Fear of Life.* New York: Macmillan, 1980.
Lowen on Oedipal conflicts and our general withholding from life—the risks of aliveness.

Lowen, Alexander, M.D. *The Language of the Body.* (originally published as *Physical Dynamics of Character Structure.*) New York: Macmillan, 1958.
Early Lowen. Lowen has written so much, so regularly, and with such impact in his area—creating a whole therapeutic approach, in effect—that it is difficult to sum up. He is one of the principal theoreticians after Reich.

Lowen, Alexander, M.D. *Love and Orgasm.* New York: Macmillan, 1975.
I find Lowen's limitations—and we all have them—more disturbing in this book than anywhere else, partly because of his emphasis on pathology, partly because of his biases, which conflict with mine.

Lowen, Alexander, M.D. *Narcissism: Denial of the True Self.* New York: Macmillan, 1983.
Image opposes self-experience and creates unreality and horror. I find this a muddy book in the general context of character structure, but others love it.

Lowen, Alexander, M.D. *Pleasure: A Creative Approach to Life.* New York: Lancer Books, 1970.

Lowen, Alexander, M.D., and Lowen, Leslie. *The Way to Vibrant Health: A Manual of Bioenergetic Exercises.* New York: Harper Colophon, 1977.
Just what it says: a collection of the most commonly used bioenergetic

exercises for moving energy and re-distributing it. They are effective for many "blocks" of energy in the voluntary musculature. For smaller scale interruptions of flow, I have found the Kum Nye exercises of Tarthang Tulku preferable.

Mahler, Margaret S., Rine, Fred, and Bergman, Anni. *The Psychological Birth of the Human Infant: Symbiosis and Individuation.* New York: Basic Books, 1975.

The result of twenty years of observation and research with normal infants, this book describes the processes by which young children learn to create boundaries and be separate.

Masters, Robert, Ph.D., and Houston, Jean Ph.D. *Listening to the Body: The Psychophysical Way to Health and Awareness.* New York: Dell, 1978.

Masters and Houston move to include the "body" in the "mind", mostly via Feldenkrais.

Masters, Robert, and Houston, Jean. *Mind Games: The Guide to Inner Space.* New York: Dell, 1972.

A classic of programmed learning exercises for the alteration of consciousness.

Miller, Roberta De Long. *Psychic Massage.* New York: Harper and Row, 1975.

Includes the energy body in touching and being touched. Some nice hints for stretching the range of your perception of touch.

Mishkin, Julie Russo, and Schill, Marta. *The Compleat Belly Dancer.* Garden City, New York: Doubleday & Company, 1973.

A full range of exercises for areas we generally leave out.

Montagu, Ashley. *Touching: The Human Significance of the Skin.* (2nd ed.) New York: Harper, 1978.

Invaluable.

Morris, Eric, and Hotchkis, Joan. *No Acting Please.* Burbank, California: Whitehouse/Spelling Publications, 1977.

"Acting is the art of creating genuine realities on a stage." (p. 1) Exercises to shake mind, emotions, and body out of a rut and into chosen movement. Morris is rather flamboyant, with a tendency to balloon.

Namgyal Rinpoche. *Body Speech and Mind.* Ottawa, Ontario: Crystal Staff Publications, 1983.

This is the best introduction I know to Tantric, or Vajrayana, Buddhism. It's a very practical, experiential approach to alteration of the bases of being, put together from talks by a Canadian teacher who was "recognised" as a Tibetan incarnation by the sixteenth Gwalma Karmapa (what *varied* realities all on one planet). English is his first language, which helps enormously.

Nam-mKhai snying po. *Mother of Knowledge: The Enlightenment of Ye-shes mTsho-rgyal.* Tarthang Tulku, trans. Berkeley, California: Dharma Publishing, 1983.

The story of one of the great Tibetan spiritual heroines. Part of the story has to do with mystical sexual union as a teaching method, but you are expected to learn from a teacher.

Ostrander, Sheila, and Schroeder, Lynn. *Psychic Discoveries Behind the Iron Curtain*. Englewood Cliffs, New Jersey: Prentice-Hall, 1970.

Padget, Desmond. *Transcendental Sensuality*. New York: Lancer Books, 1973.

Despite its suspect title, this is a rather fine introduction to simple tantra, seen as the extension and refining of sensation and perception through all the senses. Focusses on sex, but the exercises are directed to all sensory pathways and are not all sexual in intention. No direct energetic exercises.

Pagels, Heinz R. *The Cosmic Code: Quantum Physics as the Language of Nature*. New York: Simon and Schuster, 1982.

An exciting book on its subject. Unlike *The Dancing Wu Li Masters* or *The Tao of Physics* or *The Medium, the Mystic and the Physicist*, Pagels stringently denies any significance of quantum mechanics outside the world of particle physics, but (I find) is constantly and unconsciously undermining his own position. For me, this adds to the interest of the book.

Rajneesh, Bhagwan Shree. *The Book of Secrets, Vols. I-V*. New York: Harper and Row, 1974.

This is Rajneesh's commentary on the "Vigyana Bhairava Tantra"—112 methods of meditation (i.e., altering consciousness and moving energy) attributed to Shiva. Tantric but not specifically sexual.

Rajneesh, Bhagwan Shree. *Only One Sky: On the Tantric Way of Tilopa's Song of Mahamudra*. New York: E. P. Dutton, 1975.

A commentary on the classic Tibetan tantric poem. The commentary itself is tantric in orientation, that is, is oriented towards acceptance of life and being in all its aspects.

Reich, Wilhelm, M.D. *Character Analysis*. (3rd, expanded ed.) New York: Farrar, Straus & Giroux, 1967.

Introduces the then-revolutionary notion that the body reflects character and that therefore the body must be dealt with in psychotherapy. A classic, still exciting to read. Some flavour of the Young Turk.

Reich, Wilhelm. *Cosmis Superimposition: Man's Orgonotic Roots in Nature*. Orgonon, Rangeley, Maine: Wilhelm Reich Foundation, 1951.

Reich's study of the spiral form and movement in man, nature, and the cosmos. Compare to Schwenk's *Sensitive Chaos* and to Reich's own works of a slightly later period when he had begun to lose his personal ground.

Reich, Wilhelm. *The Function of the Orgasm: Sex-Economic Problems of Biological Energy*. New York: Bantam Books, 1967 (written 1926).

Another classic, which really stirred the waters at the time. The reflexive nature of orgasm. Orgasmic redistribution of energy as the "energy economy" of the body. Reich is said to have felt physically unwell if he went two days without orgasm, which may have influenced the strength of his view.

Reich, Wilhelm. *Listen, Little Man!* New York: Farrar, Straus and Giroux, 1948.

Reich talking to himself and to us privately (not originally intended for publication), trying to work out his angers and conflicts over social and personal suppression of life and flow.

Reich, Wilhelm. *The Murder of Christ: The Emotional Plague of Mankind.* New York: Farrar, Strauss and Giroux, 1953. Written June–August, 1951. Discusses the effects—social and personal—of living an armoured life: hatred of that which lives fully. Reich identifies with Christ.

Reich, Wilhelm. *Selected Writings: An Introduction to Orgonomy.* New York: Farrar, Straus and Cudahy, 1961.
Bits and pieces from practically every area of Reich's work. A good place to start a study of his work.

Reich, Wilhelm. *The Sexual Revolution: Towards Self-Governing Character Structure.* (4th ed.) New York: Farrar, Straus and Giroux, 1967. (First copyright, 1945.)
Sex and society. Social and sexual repression closely related.

Rosen, Sydney, M.D., ed. *My Voice Will Go with You: The Teaching Tales of Milton H. Erickson, M.D.* (includes commentaries by Rosen). New York: W. W. Norton & Company, 1982.
The most approachable book there is on Erickson's teaching through stories. The stories are great, too.

Rosenberg, Jack Lee. *Total Orgasm.* New York: Random House, 1973. Catchy title. An admirable introduction to bioenergetic exercises which effect energy flow and charge, specifically to increase sexual pleasure. Rosenberg discusses union as *confluence* and has a chapter on spirituality and orgasm. He doesn't deal with how to influence energy flow directly, though, of course, all the exercises are intended to affect charge, flow, and surrender.

Rush, Anne Kent. *Getting Clear: Body Work for Women.* New York: Random House, 1973.
One of the first books for women on reclaiming their physical beings.

Schwarz, Jack. *Human Energy Systems.* New York: E. P. Dutton, 1980. Another approach to direct perception of human energies—and what to do about it. Schwarz is famous for his voluntary control over physical/energetic processes.

Schwartz-Salant, Nathan. "Archetypal Factors Underlying Sexual Acting Out in the Transference/Countertransference Process." *Chiron*, 1984. A Jungian approaching issues of energetic union from his own experience and within a Jungian vocabulary.

Schwenk, Theodor. *Sensitive Chaos: The Creation of Flowing Forms in Water and Air.* New York: Schocken Books, 1978. (First published, 1965.)
Spirals and waves, waves and spirals, everywhere in form and movement. Striking book, especially for the pictures. Compare Young's *Reflexive Universe*, Tohei on aikido (where the spiral and the wave are embodied), and Reich on orgone in the individual and the cosmos (*Cosmic Superimposition*).

Smith, David. *The East/West Exercise Book.* New York: McGraw-Hill,

1976.
Many exercises that can be explored from the perspective of attention and presence. All of them have effects on energy distribution and emotional "flavour" of being, as well as on physical strength, flexibility, and tone.

Spolin, Viola. *Improvisation for the Theater: A Handbook of Teaching and Directing Techniques.* Evanston, Illinois: Northwestern University Press, 1963.
A basic text on the creation of realities through physical imagination. Spolin's methods directly influenced some of the most creative and convincing actors of the current crop (e.g., Alan Arkin, Nichols and May).

Stevens, John O. *Awareness: Exploring, Experimenting, Experiencing.* Lafayette, California: Real People Press, 1971.
Lots and lots of Gestalt exercises for noticing what's happening inside and outside. Could easily be an introductory acting text. Or a Western meditation similar to vipassana.

Swami Jyotirmayanda. *Meditate the Tantric Yoga Way.* New York: E. P. Dutton, 1973.
Meditations with sound and visualisation involving the major chakras (energy centres) in the body. A nonsexual, Indian approach, which is nevertheless intended to arouse *shakti* (the primal energy of being, regarded as female) and move to union with it.

Tarthang Tulku. *Kum Nye Relaxation, vols. I-II.* Berkeley, California: Dharma Publishing, 1978.
Far and away the most effective and powerful exercises collected anywhere (that I know of, in English) for the balancing and integrating, stimulating and transforming of energies. The exercises were developed by Tarthang Tulku over a period of years working with Western students; they are based on tantra and Tibetan medicine. I use them all the time myself and with others. I usually recommend that in the beginning people make expressive sounds as part of the exercises and let silence come gradually.

Thie, John F., D.C. *Touch for Health.* (Revised ed.) Marina del Rey, California: DeVorss and Company, 1979.
This is a practical introduction to applied kinesiology and acupressure as a form of treatment for physical and mental discomforts. I see it as a fine way to explore the intelligence of the body and its willingness to communicate meaningfully, e.g., through muscle-testing. In fact, muscle-testing can be used "hypnotically"—without obvious alterations of consciousness—to communicate directly with the unconscious mind.

Thirleby, Ashley. *Tantra: The Key to Sexual Power and Pleasure.* New York: Dell, 1978.
Another suspect title on a very usable book (out-of-print, unfortunately). Visualisation, sound, concentration in exercises to increase energy level. The increased charge can be used for sexual pleasure, but Thirleby is equally interested in collecting sexual energy and channel-

ling it to other goals. Does make the false assumptions, however, that most people know how to charge themselves—sexually or otherwise.

Toben, Bob, and Wolf, Fred Alan. *Space-Time and Beyond: Toward an Explanation of the Unexplainable.* (New ed.) New York: E. P. Dutton, 1982.
A pleasant way to loosen assumptions about how things are and can be.

Tohei, Koichi. *Book of Ki: Co-ordinating Mind and Body in Daily Life.* Tokyo: Japan Publications, 1976.
One of the few books related to a martial art (aikido) that offers something helpful to the uninformed reader. Better yet, try *ki* practice in aikido, t'ai chi, or some other martial art with emphasis on energy in movement.

Watzlawick, Paul. *How Real Is Real? Confusion, Disinformation, Communication: An Anecdotal Introduction to Communications Theory.* New York: Random House, 1976.
Absolutely splendid. Playful, knowledgeable, approachable.

Watzlawick, Paul. *The Language of Change: Elements of Therapeutic Communication.* New York: Basic Books, 1978.
A lucid, brilliant discussion of how language makes meaning and how to alter the attitudinal realities we hold in metaphor.

Wilbur, Ken. *No Boundary: Eastern and Western Approaches to Personal Growth.* Boulder, Colorado: Shambhala, 1981.
Wilbur is one of the most prolific of the current theoreticians of transpersonal psychology. Here his discussion of the relativity of boundaries is very helpful.

Wilson, Robert Anton. *Prometheus Rising.* Phoenix, Arizona: Falcon Press, 1983.
Riding the line between speculative fiction and flaky thinking in a very productive and "Ericksonian" way, Wilson sets out to dislodge assumptions about what is and what we perceive. Exercises for altering your reality.

Windels, Jenny. *Eutonie mit Kindern.* München: Kösel-Verlag, 1984.
Original in Dutch, no English available yet. This lovely book by a leading student of Gerda Alexander is full of exercises that support awareness in the body and integration of "self" and "body". Many of them develop presence and contactfulness. Discussion of their use with children.

Young, Arthur M. *The Reflexive Universe: Evolution of Consciousness.* (No city given): Delacorte Press, 1976.

Zeig, Jeffrey K., Ph.D., ed. *A Teaching Seminar with Milton H. Erickson, M.D.* New York: Brunner/Mazel, 1980.
A whole lot of Erickson direct from transcript. If you know what Erickson sounds like (there are tapes available), you can alter your state of consciousness and hear it right off the page as you read.

Zukav, Gary. *The Dancing Wu Li Masters: An Overview of the New Physics.* New York: William Morrow, 1979.
Story of the origins and continuation of the radical change in our understanding of how things are.

About the Author

Julie Henderson, Ph.D., has combined body-oriented psychotherapy, Ericksonian hypnotherapy, and 20 years of study with Tibetan high lamas into a form of personal work and training that emphasizes the direct passage to pleasure and well-being. She calls this work *Zapchen*, from a Tibetan word that suggests a salubrious, mind-changing naughtiness.

She is widely known for her unrehearsed, once-upon-a-time stories. For many years, with Sydney Australia as her base, Ms. Henderson traveled internationally conducting seminars and classes in bodywork, energetics, and story-telling. She was the first president of the Australian Association of Somatic Psychotherapists. She teaches with the approval and at the request of her Tibetan teachers. At their suggestion, she has returned from Australia to live and work in her native U.S.

Julie Henderson is also the author of *Embodying Well-Being: How to Feel as Good as You Can in Spite of Everything.*

She welcomes comments and inquiries.

E-mail: Zapchenma@aol.com
Web page: http://members.aol.com/zapchenma/